W9-BDZ-589

Praise for *The Fatigue Solution*

"Dr. Eva Cwynar takes a woman's complaint of fatigue seriously. Drawing on her work as an endocrinologist, she outlines an eight-step solution for women that is prescriptive, practical, and empowering."

— **Marie Savard M.D.**, women's health expert, author,
and ABC News medical contributor

"Creating a schedule is one thing; keeping up with it is another.
The Fatigue Solution *is the key to maintaining the energy necessary to accomplish it all. My compliments to Dr. Cwynar."*

— **Lyn Davis Lear, Ph.D.**, philanthropist and political activist

"The entertainment business is extremely draining on all levels. We work long hours under difficult circumstances. ***The Fatigue Solution*** *offers an easy program for excellent results. Everyone can benefit from the simple lifestyle changes Dr. Cwynar suggests."*

— **Morgan Fairchild**, actress and activist

"As an Olympic-level athlete, I have to be at my best at all times. Reading ***The Fatigue Solution*** *has helped me to achieve that goal. Dr. Cwynar's advice, from how to maintain maximum energy levels to how to deal with the stress of intense competition, has proved invaluable. She's a champion in my book!"*

— **Leslie Morse**, international equestrian champion

*"**The Fatigue Solution** has the medical recipe for all the demands my position holds. Bravo Dr. Cwynar!"*

— **Sylvia Bongo**, first lady of Gabon, Africa

"I was feeling fatigued almost every day, and now I can actually feel my vitality getting stronger every day. Many thanks, Dr. Cwynar!"

— **Ricki Lake**, talk show host, actress, and author

"Hormone imbalance can wreak havoc on your body. Dr. Cwynar has been able to help me, and this book will be able to help you, too. She helped me to understand the problem as well as the solution. I highly recommend ***The Fatigue Solution.****"*

— **Dr. Andrea Rich**, ex vice chancellor emeritus UCLA,
president-director of Los Angeles County Museum of Arts (Retired)

the
fatigue
solution

the
fatigue
solution

Increase Your Energy in Eight Easy Steps

Eva Cwynar, M.D.
with Sharyn Kolberg

HAY HOUSE, INC.
Carlsbad, California • New York City
London • Sydney • Johannesburg
Vancouver • Hong Kong • New Delhi

Published and distributed in the United States by: Hay House, Inc.: www.hayhouse.com • *Published and distributed in Australia by:* Hay House Australia Pty. Ltd.: www.hayhouse.com.au • *Published and distributed in the United Kingdom by:* Hay House UK, Ltd.: www.hayhouse.co.uk • *Published and distributed in the Republic of South Africa by:* Hay House SA (Pty), Ltd.: www.hayhouse.co.za • *Distributed in Canada by:* Raincoast: www.raincoast.com • *Published in India by:* Hay House Publishers India: www.hayhouse.co.in

Design: Julie Davison

Library of Congress Cataloging-in-Publication Data

Cwynar, Eva
  The fatigue solution : increase your energy in eight easy steps / Eva Cwynar, Sharyn Kolberg.
     p. cm.
  Includes bibliographical references.
  ISBN 978-1-4019-3163-6 (hardback)
  1. Fatigue--Alternative treatment. 2. Women--Health and hygiene. 3. Nutrition. I. Kolberg, Sharyn. II. Title.
  RB150.F37C89 2012
  616'.0478--dc23
                                            2011040365

Hardcover ISBN: 978-1-4019-3163-6
Digital ISBN: 978-1-4019-3165-0

15 14 13 12   4 3 2 1
1st edition, March 2012

Printed in the United States of America

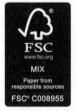

I dedicate this book to my daughters, Danielle and Nicole Kohut. You are my purpose in life. Your inspiration is limitless. Always be strong, embrace love, and above all, enjoy life!

Contents

Foreword

My children were two and three years old when I started *Desperate Housewives.* I had a wonderful husband, two perfect children, and the best job I could ever hope for. I was even in a movie that was getting a lot of attention; in short, all my dreams were coming true. Except I was tired—I am talking algebra-class tired—you know, where you put your head down on any surface and fall asleep drooling? Time passed, and I went from tired to exhausted to fatigued, chronically fatigued. My immune system was so compromised that every two or three days I was sick with a sore throat or a slight fever. I went to chiropractors, homeopaths, internists, gynecologists, GPs, and gastroenterologists. One doctor put me on estrogen, progesterone, and testosterone. I stopped eating dairy; I stopped eating wheat; I stopped eating sugar; I just plain stopped eating. Nothing worked. I began to doubt my own symptoms and started to blame myself for feeling so terrible.

Then I found Dr. Cwynar and everything changed. She sat me down in her office and talked to me for an hour. She listened, she questioned, and she took my symptoms seriously. She looked me in the eye and said, "It's okay, we are going to figure this out and you *will* feel better." I wasn't just a patient and she wasn't just another doctor; we were a team and she was dedicated to improving my health. She put me through a battery of tests (many of the ones she recommends in this book) checking for vitamin deficiencies, hormone levels, cortisol levels, and digestive track efficiency. Everything. I mean *everything.*

It worked. Dr. Cwynar, with her comprehensive approach, was able to get me the sleep I needed, the proper hormones for my body, and the supplements to support my health. It has not only transformed my day-to-day experience but also allowed me to be hopeful for the future. I have a core of energy that I haven't had since before my two children were born.

If fatigue is an issue for you, you will find yourself in this book. Even if it takes until Chapter 4 or 5 for you to suddenly say "Aha! That's what is going on with me!" As you continue to read you'll realize that most conditions overlap and nothing stands alone. So the whole book becomes very pertinent. *The Fatigue Solution* gives you simple yet powerful tools to help you and your doctor figure it all out. Or to realize that perhaps it is time you find a new doctor.

Dr. Cwynar empowers you to take charge of your health and gives you the information and tools to make a difference. The most important message of this book is that no matter how hectic or demanding your lifestyle or what stage of life you are in, you don't have to settle for feeling bad. Fatigue is not inevitable. You deserve to feel better. And you can feel better—you can even feel great.

— Felicity Huffman, television and film actress

Introduction

I wrote this book to help you get the "F" word out of your life. You know what I'm talking about. Maybe you've lost that lust for life you had when you were younger, and you wonder why it's gone. Maybe it's that you want to "bring the sexy back" into your life but you just don't know how to reignite that flame of desire. Maybe you want to find a way to relieve some of the stress in your life—the stress that's been keeping you anxious all day and preventing you from getting a good night's sleep.

Or maybe you're just tired of being tired all the time, and you're determined to get the "F" word—fatigue—out of your life once and for all.

Whatever your reasons, you'll be glad you picked up this book.

Women all over the world have similar concerns. I hear it over and over again from the women who come to me for help, women who feel overwhelmed and undertreated, women who are looking for ways to take control of their lives and their health. Women who have busy lives and are looking for real solutions—simple steps they can fit into their daily routines. Women who are just like me.

You Don't Have to Take It Anymore

Too many women are willing to accept that the older they get, the less energy they will have. The myth that has been perpetuated by doctors and patients alike is that there's nothing you can do about most of the problems associated with getting older. You have aches and pains? That's to be expected. You're putting on weight? That's to be expected. You're losing your hair? That's to be expected. You're losing interest in sex? Of course; you're getting older.

I am here to tell you that it is unacceptable to view any of these things as inevitable consequences of aging. I've helped grateful women around the world not only boost their energy levels but also get back the enthusiasm they had for life when they were younger. After successfully integrating the Fatigue Solution program into her life, one patient felt so different that it was noticeable to everyone around her. Her friend even remarked about how she must be thrilled by her "new" self. To which my patient replied, *"No, this is the old me. I got the old me back, and that's what I really wanted."*

That's what I always expect to hear from my patients, and that's what I want for you. Obviously, I can't treat every woman in the world. That's why I wrote this book. I wanted to teach as many women as possible these eight easy steps, so they can reenergize and revitalize their own lives, and feel empowered to take control of their own health and their own futures.

It's All about the Hormones

Most of my patients have been referred to me by friends or family members whose lives have been changed by learning about the eight essential steps to energy revitalization that are laid out in this book. When they come to my office, many of them are not even quite sure that I'm an M.D. They might think I'm a family practitioner, a nutritionist, or a homeopath. But they come to me because they are at their wits' end. They've seen several other doctors, and they don't know where else to turn. I hear it over and over again: "You're my last resort. If you can't help me, I'll just crawl into a cave somewhere and eat my way into old age." They feel that they have no other options left.

What I am is an endocrinologist—a hormone specialist—which means that I help women (and men) deal with the effects of hormones on the body, both inside *and* outside. An endocrinologist is a physician who has completed four years of medical school and then three years of training in internal medicine and then an additional two years studying hormones. Essentially, endocrinologists have twice the amount of training of most other physicians, with a particular focus on hormones and metabolism.

We are currently facing a nationwide shortage of endocrinologists, with approximately 2,400 practicing in the United States. These specialists, most of whom are in New York and California, focus on treating adults. That's a relatively small number when compared to most other medical specialties. That means there are very few of us who have the training and specialized knowledge to fully understand hormones—what they do in the body and how they do what they do—and I am proud to be among that small group of medical specialists.

Hormones are powerful chemical messengers that are produced by a number of different glands, circulate through the bloodstream, and generate a wide range of biological responses. Hormones affect both your physical and emotional well-being. If you're happy or sad, depressed or elated, or angry or tired; if you feel hungry or sleepy or sexy, your body is responding to hormones.

Some doctors (and patients) don't take fatigue seriously. But it is a real disease. It has its own International Classification of Diseases (ICD-9) code. The ICD-9 is a listing of all diseases so that they can be billed for insurance reimbursement.

If you're chronically fatigued, chances are it's because of hormones. If you're experiencing unexplained weight gain, hair loss, or dry skin, chances are it's because of hormones. If you look in the mirror and notice your skin looking older than it did yesterday, chances are it's because of hormones. If you can get your hormones rebalanced, you can also turn back the clock, both internally and externally. When your hormones run as they should, your energy, youth, and overall health can be restored.

From the Bush to Beverly Hills—
A World View of Medicine

Medicine is in my blood. My mother is a physician who devotes her life to the underprivileged children of the South Bronx. It's part of my identity and why I've spent years trying to better understand who I am to better help my patients understand who they are . . . and who they can be.

Many of my patients come to me in a state of frustration because they don't understand what's happening to them, and other doctors can't seem to help them. I recently had a patient who flew in from Florida, and when I asked why she had flown all the way to Los Angeles, she said, "Because I described my symptoms for my doctor, and he just tuned me out. I told him I wanted my thyroid checked, and he just ignored me. When I told him I just didn't feel like myself, I could tell he wasn't listening to what I was saying." I hear this all the time. If a symptom is not site specific (e.g., stomachache, chest pain), doctors don't know what to do about it. In the Western world, physicians are taught how to treat life and death and disease almost as individual components, not as part of a larger picture.

I look at medicine with a much broader perspective. By the time I was 30, I had traveled to more than 100 countries, and I have continued my travels throughout my life in my quest to find out how indigenous peoples deal, both medically and philosophically, with the issues and ills they face. I've traveled throughout the entire continent of South America and lived there for a year to learn about native Indian cultures and the tremendous amount of medicinal herbs that come from this continent. I went to Australia to learn about Aborigines' survival habits. I climbed Mt. Kilimanjaro with my husband on our honeymoon to see how people responded to the extreme changes in climate and altitude, from tropics to frozen weather at 19,342 feet above sea level. (My husband wasn't expecting to hear "Not tonight dear, I can hardly breathe" on his honeymoon!) I've been to many parts of Asia to learn about meditation as well as local medicinal customs with the monks; I've also visited such out-of-the-way destinations as Burma, Mongolia, and Tibet, where I gathered information on how these cultures deal with issues of aging and fatigue.

In the summer of 2011, I traveled to Africa to study with the tribal doctors of the pygmies of Gabon. I was able to do this only by invitation of the president of Gabon, as these tribes are isolated and want to remain that way. I was thrilled to be one of the very few people to have the privilege of traveling into the thick of the jungle, by small plane, helicopter, and canoe, to spend time with these fascinating people, especially with their tribal doctors.

I've been to all regions of Africa to study with tribal doctors and shamans. What I found most interesting was that, despite the fact that Zambia has more than 70 tribal languages, Botswana has more than 30, and South Africa has hundreds more, I couldn't find a word among them that translated into *fatigue*. Perhaps they don't experience fatigue in the way that we do, and therefore don't have a word for it.

Western society is beginning to incorporate some "alternative medicine" into its practices—mostly Chinese herbs and acupuncture. But we've ignored the traditions from the land where humanity started and what we can learn from the *sangoma,* the African tribal healers. We rarely study the medicine that comes from that part of the world, and yet it's been around almost since the birth of mankind. The most important lesson I have learned from their practices is that they don't just give their patients potions and powders and send them on their way. They look at everything that's going on in their lives—at their daily routines, their relationships with family and friends. So, depending on their illness, a patient might be given medicine plus instructions on what time to get up in the morning, what kinds of food he must eat, and how he must treat his mother-in-law. It's all a part of the healing process.

So now when I ask personal and sometimes embarrassing questions of my patients, I explain that it's not because I'm intruding into their private lives. I ask questions because unless I understand how they function in their family, in their job, in their travels, and in their daily life, I can't understand what's going on with them hormonally. It's not just the body that's involved; it's everything in their lives that led them to me.

I believe that by studying the ancient cultures, by studying the best of what has survived for thousands of years, we can enlighten our futures. Our ancestors have much to teach us; we cannot afford to ignore these teachings if we want to survive.

> " . . . our search for a future that works keeps
> spiraling back to an ancient connection between
> ourselves and the earth, an interconnectedness that
> ancient cultures have never abandoned."
>
> —HELENA NORBERG-HODGE,
> FOUNDER OF THE INTERNATIONAL
> SOCIETY FOR ECOLOGY AND CULTURE

I Am Woman . . .

I believe that women can do it all (although maybe not all at once) because we are incredible multitaskers. I know it is possible because I do it every day. As you read this book, you will discover that it is not only about your fighting fatigue—it's my story, too. There have been times when I was not in the best of health, and I needed to do something about it. I needed a way to get more energy into my life and to sustain it for as long as possible. After all, I am a wife, a mother, a daughter, and a doctor. Needless to say, my life is exceedingly hectic.

My point is that if I can survive all this and do it all reasonably well, that alone should make me something of an expert in the subject of energy. My hectic life, which is just like a million other hectic lives, is the reason I developed the Fatigue Solution program. I don't have time to be tired all the time; I don't want to be tired all the time; and for the sake of my husband, my children, and myself, I can't be tired all the time. The more I thought about it, the more I realized there were areas of my life I could definitely improve to get my energy back, and they became the eight steps of this program. They had to be simple; they had to be doable; they had to improve the quality of my life. As you read my story, you will see that when my life got off track, I got my energy (and my life) back by following the Fatigue Solution program. And you can, too.

The Eight Easy Steps

Although many of the women who come to me complaining of fatigue are in their late 30s and older, it's never too early (or too late) to start the Fatigue Solution program. When we're in our 20s, our hormones are usually strong and plentiful. However, hormones start to diminish in both quantity and quality by the time we reach our 30s. That's when we need to start preparing ourselves for the aging process. By the time we're in our 40s or 50s, ingrained habits are difficult to break.

This book will show you how to maintain your energy and vitality. You'll learn how your hormones create a delicate balance throughout your body's systems and how, when some of those hormones are out of balance, it can throw your overall health way off course and sap your energy resources. You'll also learn what energy is all about—how it is produced in the body and what we need to do to keep it going throughout our busy, demanding lives. Then you'll discover the eight essential metabolically and scientifically based steps to restoring your personal power, your health, your longevity, and your quality of life. Each of these steps is important on its own, but they all work together to restore and repair your energy resources:

❖ **Step #1. Feed Your Energy Furnace:** Red meat, anyone? Whole milk? Omelets made with egg whites *and* yolks? The first step to revitalization is knowing which foods—including, surprisingly, the ones just mentioned—fuel your energy furnace and ensure a healthier, more vital future. (In Appendix I, you'll be introduced to "Dr. Eva's Energy/Fuel Matrix," a protein-based way of eating that will get your eating habits on track and fuel your body's energy needs.)

❖ **Step #2. Get Your Gut in Shape:** The foods you eat and your lifestyle in general can be causing your body a great deal of stress. It may seem a little odd, but the truth is that your gastrointestinal tract is tied into your energy levels, and simply by clearing out toxins, you can help rejuvenate your entire system. You don't have to be a fanatic; there are simple things you can do to keep your body free of pollutants and toxins.

❖ **Step #3. Improve Your Sleep Habits:** No doubt about it: sleep deprivation equals energy depletion. It's the quality of sleep that counts (getting up even once a night to pee is one time too many) if you want to make it through the day at the top of your game. The truth is that getting the right type of sleep is more important than just going to bed. Discover the step-by-step guidelines for creating physical, mental, and emotional calm and healthy sleeping schedules to keep your hormones balanced and your energy flowing.

❖ **Step #4. Supercharge Your Sexuality:** A good sex life increases overall energy. Sex does a body good; it releases endorphins and revs up your metabolism. But as with sleep, it's the quality of your sex life that makes the difference. You may want to turn to this chapter first . . . and that's okay. It can be a great way to revitalize your relationship and get the juices flowing in the rest of your life!

❖ **Step #5. Move Your Body and Boost Your Metabolism:** Simply put, exercise gives you energy. It helps you lose weight, keeps your heart healthy, and lessens depression. There are specific exercises, however, that are designed to increase energy output throughout the day. This chapter will also reveal the secret "sexiness" of exercise—there's something about a sweaty woman after a workout that turns a man on and boosts his metabolism as well as yours. There are plenty of ways to exercise without having to step on a treadmill (for example, boxing releases aggression along with a whole lot of calories). Learn quick techniques to promote physical health between phone calls or business meetings, and things to do at your desk that pay off with bursts of burned calories. It's easy to get the maximum benefits with these fun exercise options.

❖ **Step #6. Check Your Thyroid:** Current estimates show that millions of Americans have some type of thyroid condition; however, millions more have a thyroid condition and don't know it. How much energy and stamina you have on a daily basis is directly related to the thyroid hormone. The vast majority with thyroid conditions are hypothyroid, which means they have an underfunctioning, slow, or sluggish thyroid. When women are run-down and overweight, many automatically assume they are having thyroid problems. For some women, that is indeed the case. For others it is not. It's important to know how you can find out if your thyroid is doing its job and how to keep it working efficiently.

❖ **Step #7. Prepare Yourself for "That Time of the Month":** Out-of-control hormones can spin you out of control every month if you're not careful. However, there are several steps (such as increasing certain B vitamins and decreasing caffeine consumption), as well as herbs and supplements you can take before, during, and after that time of the month to keep from suffering debilitating energy loss. Women who are experiencing perimenopause and menopause will also find special sections on retaining and maintaining energy reserves as they get older.

❖ **Step #8. Have Yourself Tested:** There are many different diagnostic tests available today. Some must be done in a doctor's office and some you can do at home. Your doctor may not even know about some of these tests—not every doctor knows what cutting-edge medicine has to offer these days. They will tell you if you are deficient in certain trace minerals and other micronutrients or if you have neurotransmitter imbalances that are contributing to the problems of energy depletion and fatigue. The tests recommended in this chapter will quickly let you know what and how much you need to get your body back on track.

As you will hear from many of my patients throughout this book, it is definitely possible to get back to the "you" you used to be. If you've lost that feeling of excitement and anticipation about what might happen tomorrow, don't you want it back again? At what point is "just getting through the day" not okay anymore?

Why not leap into the rest of your life? There's no reason to accept what others may see as an inevitable slowdown when following the Fatigue Solution program can help you regain mental clarity, restore your vitality, and reclaim your life.

CHAPTER 1

The Quality
of Your Life

I once treated a working mother who was suffering from severe fatigue, an almost total lack of energy, a low sex drive, and chronic infections after the birth of her second child. She was a busy professional and was worried that her constant tiredness would affect her ability to do her job and care for her family. Her concentration and memory were unreliable at best. Sleep, what little she got, never refreshed her. She had no interest in having sex with her husband. Typically she crawled into bed around 7:00 P.M., leaving her children to be cared for by others. Internists, ob-gyns, infectious disease specialists, gastroenterologists, and ear, nose, and throat doctors were all mystified by her run-down condition. Her blood and saliva were tested for vitamin, mineral, and hormone levels, and the results showed a multitude of nutrient deficiencies and hormone imbalances. With the help of the nutritionist in my office, I started her on an energy-specific diet to support her body's systems and help them absorb more nutrients while giving her supplements to help replenish the vitamins and minerals her body lacked. I also adjusted her hormones. Within two months, she felt more focused and could now stay awake in the evenings after work. Most encouraging, her immune system was strong enough to resist the flu bug running through her office. After five months, I was thrilled to learn that her overall energy level had increased dramatically and, as an added benefit, her sex drive had revived.

Why was this case so special? Because this patient I'd healed was me, Dr. Eva Cwynar.

1

Every day, all over the world, millions of women just like me are grappling with many of these same mind and body issues, and more: low sex drive, weight gain, sexual dissatisfaction, chronic stress, anxiety, hormonal mood imbalances, infertility, poor sleep, lack of concentration, PMS, perimenopause and menopause complications, and most especially, an overriding feeling of inexplicable fatigue. Well, it's time to take the "F" word out of our lives! This book will show you how you can go from fatigued to fabulous by helping you identify and understand the potential source of your vexing health conditions, no matter what your age. It is a 21st-century woman's health guide for generating physical and emotional strength, balancing hormones, reclaiming sexual vitality, and restoring energy.

Women travel from all over to see me with the same kinds of complaints I suffered several years ago. But their biggest complaint, the one that I hear over and over again in these times of overscheduled, overstressed, and overstimulated lives, is that they are more than just tired. They're more tired than they've ever been. They have lost the energy they used to have, and they want it back again. Women ranging in age from their 30s to their 70s plead with me to help them regain that core inner flame that has now become an ember barely burning.

Dealing with the Energy Crisis

Women often tell me that they never had energy problems when they were 20; that they could work all day and party all night and bounce right back into the swing of things. I can't promise that after you read this book you will be as resilient you were at 20. We can't totally ignore the fact that we're aging. As we age, it takes more time, more effort, and more patience to keep energy levels high. But the eight simple steps laid out in this book will help you get the results you want.

Unfortunately, women frequently come to see me upset by all the doctors they've seen who don't acknowledge that they have legitimate complaints and who dismiss the fact that they have no energy. I want you to get a second, third, or even tenth opinion (or until you get a satisfactory answer). I believe that you know your body better than anyone else. You owe it to yourself to keep searching when you know there is something wrong with you. What you're feeling is real. I want you to fight to reclaim your energy—to say that it's not just that you're aging or you've got children or you've been working too hard. Until the 1980s, many doctors discounted women's complaints about menopause. In fact, nobody talked about it; most women just accepted the way they felt and listened to doctors who told them there was nothing to be done about it. Those doctors were wrong (as you'll find out in Chapter 8); and today, women have many options to help them deal with the symptoms of menopause.

The same thing is happening with the women's "energy crisis" that is occurring today. Women no longer accept "experts" saying, "Sorry, nothing's wrong with you—you're just getting older."

I get the same comment from my patients over and over again: "My God! Where do you get your energy?" Patients e-mail me over the weekend and are shocked when I e-mail them right back. They say, "I didn't think you'd answer until Monday. I can't believe you're still working!" I figure if I can do it, everyone else can, too. I do it with passion and enthusiasm. But I had to go through my own battle with fatigue and work my way out of it before I truly understood that I didn't just have to accept what was happening to my emotional and physical being.

That's what *The Fatigue Solution* is all about: taking charge of your life so that you can recharge your life. Will it take some effort? Of course it will; everything worthwhile takes some effort. Will it happen overnight? No it won't. It's taken a fair amount of time to wear your systems down, and you'll need to give them time to build up again. If you really want to live a healthy, balanced life, especially as you get older, whether you're dealing with money or your personal relationships or your work life, seldom are there quick fixes. It can take many months and sometimes years to find a mate, to figure out what your career is going to be, or to write a book. If you want a more energetic life, you've got to make a commitment to yourself. You have to be willing to care about yourself. If you're not prepared to take that responsibility, to say, "This is my life and I have to be good to my body every day," then you are missing the true enjoyment that life can give you. When you do take that responsibility, you allow your body to work the way it is supposed to work, to function at its highest capacity, and to add vital, energetic years to your life.

Something So Simple

When Polly came into my office, she looked as if the weight of the world was on her shoulders. Her hair was a dull shade of brown; there was no twinkle in her eyes. She had a history of hypoglycemia (low blood sugar). She, like everyone else I know, had a busy life. She worked part-time in her husband's business and had a son in kindergarten and a two-year-old at home. She was tired.

She immediately started talking to me about estrogen and progesterone and hormone replacement. She was sure she was going through perimenopause. She was hoping that I would prescribe her medication that would, as she put it, bring her back to life.

"Wait a minute," I said. "Let's not jump to conclusions. First, let me ask you a very important question. What did you have for breakfast?"

Polly looked at me strangely but answered my question. "Oatmeal and some cut-up fruit."

That one statement gave me my first clue as to one possible reason Polly might be so tired. This is actually what I love about my life's work. Like doctors everywhere, I have been trained in saving people's lives and preventing disease, but my focus is also on preserving quality of life. And for me, that means starting with the basics of a patient's lifestyle and moving on from there.

Endocrinologists are trained to think in terms of the domino effect. We think about how one hormone in one part of the body can signal another part of the body to respond in a particular manner, and how small changes can make big differences. Understanding the why helps us get to the what.

I'm an energy specialist; it's my job to figure out why my patients are so tired and what we can do to get them reenergized, revitalized, and restored to their former selves.

So when I asked Polly what she ate for breakfast, I wasn't just being curious. When she told me her morning meal was usually oatmeal and some fruit, I knew we had found the starting line on her road to rejuvenation. Of course, I would run some tests to measure her hormone levels, but in the meantime, I suggested it might be lack of protein in her diet at the start of the day that was causing her fatigue. I recommended she add yogurt to her bowl of fruit or substitute a couple of hard-boiled eggs for her oatmeal. Something as simple as adding protein to breakfast can make an extreme difference in a patient's quality of life. Actually, everything you do can make a difference in your life—either positive or negative. The food you eat, whether or not you exercise, how much sleep you get—they all make a difference, and the best part is that the changes you make don't have to be dramatic or radical.

In fact, this whole book and the Fatigue Solution program are designed to help you make simple changes that will make a world of difference. These are things that everybody can do. It doesn't matter how old you are or what shape you're in. The recommendations in this book are achievable, fit into virtually every woman's lifestyle, and can even be fun! I'm not asking you to go on a restrictive never-eat-a-burger-again diet. In fact, I want you to eat more protein (including red meat) than you probably eat now. And I want you to eat more often. You can do that, can't you? And in terms of exercise, I don't insist that you go to the gym (although I certainly don't discourage it). If you don't have the time or the money for a class or a trainer, I'll show you how just getting out of bed can be an exercise in itself.

Getting Your House in Order

I said in the introduction that I couldn't find a word for fatigue in African tribal languages. Maybe that's because they don't have time for fatigue; they're too busy trying to survive. Of course, they get tired and experience physical exhaustion. Many of their everyday lives (and the lives of people in many third world countries as well) are more difficult than we can imagine. Often what we in the Western world experience as fatigue is very different than the kind of exhaustion they experience. Too often, we are burning too many candles at both ends. We are brought up to believe that we can have it all, and we try to have it all at once. We are so busy "doing" everything in our lives that we are too tired to really live.

Remember, too, that there are lots of ways to bring energy into your life. When interviewing women in China, the incidence of fatigue appears to be rising (their mothers never complained about being tired; now these women do). They have found that when they get tired, they get energized by meeting new people. When Americans, like my family and me, came into their village, they practically glowed with excitement and happily asked us questions about the world we lived in, or what we thought about their world, or just made pleasant conversation. They had no other agenda; they were not looking for a mate or a handout or anything other than the good feeling they got by making a friend out of someone who had been a stranger.

You don't have to go to China to feel that kind of bond with people. In the Jewish faith, it is tradition to invite a stranger or someone in need to dinner on the Sabbath and on special holidays. As with many other ethnicities, Jewish family get-togethers are a way of life. Being with family can bring a feeling of joy and connection that increases the energy quotient in your life.

Remember that everything you do, from the moment you wake up in the morning to the moment you fall asleep at night, is going to affect your life, your health, and your energy levels. Everything. What you eat (and what you don't), what time you go to sleep, how much and how well you sleep, how you respond to things emotionally. Your movement or lack of it, your actions, your choice of profession, your choice of lover, spouse, or mate.

I have patients who come into my office and tell me, "I've been dieting for weeks, and I haven't lost a pound. I don't understand it." When I question them about what else is going on in their lives, I find out that they've been incredibly busy at work, they haven't exercised in months, they're in the midst of a divorce, and they're sleeping only about four hours a night. But they're eating a few fewer calories a day and expecting the body to respond the way they want it to. News flash: nature just doesn't work that way. If you want to get your house in order, you've got to get your *whole* house in order.

The Energy Influencers: Hormones and Neurotransmitters

Utter this sentence in a crowded room: "I feel like I have no energy these days," and it's guaranteed that 90 percent of the women in the room will answer, "I know just what you mean." The problem is, most of us don't really understand what energy is, where it comes from, how it's produced in the body, and most important, how we lost the energy we once had and how to get it back.

Energy loss can be caused by a variety of factors. Fatigue is often a lot more complicated than not eating enough fruit or not getting the proper exercise. If you're going to talk about energy or the lack thereof, you've got to talk about hormones and the glands that produce them, also known as the endocrine system.

The endocrine system influences almost everything that goes on within our bodies, from sexual function and reproductive processes to the regulation of growth, mood, and metabolism. The endocrine system is made up of glands, groups of cells that produce and secrete chemicals known as hormones, or messengers that transfer information and instructions from one set of cells to another. The major glands of the endocrine system are the hypothalamus, pituitary, thyroid, parathyroids, adrenals, pineal body, and the reproductive organs (ovaries and testes). The pancreas is also a part of this system; it has a role in hormone production as well as in digestion.

When your energy is low, the endocrine system jumps into action. The thyroid and adrenal glands produce hormones that give you an extra energy boost. However, it can be an anxiety-producing, frenetic kind of energy that does not do a body good. Yes, it will help you get through the day, but it will stress your mind and your body, which will eventually lead to more fatigue. Hormones send messages to your muscles (the main storage area for glucose) saying, "911! Emergency! Give up your sugar or else!" The muscles sacrifice the glucose and become depleted to save other cells throughout the body. And that's when we crash, burn, and become exhausted.

Hormones can create chaos in your body, both internally and externally. We all know the joke: "I'm just hormonal." It's not a joke. Hormone imbalance can cause weight gain, lack of sex drive, dry skin, hair loss, and the kind of fatigue that feels like no amount of sleep could ever make it go away. Hormones are also one of the primary causes of accelerated aging. From the inside out, suddenly you are no longer the person you have always known. While you (and your doctor) may chalk it up to growing older, I know differently.

Tuning In to Hormonal Signals

When hormones are released, they circulate through your bloodstream and come in contact with all your cells. However, only certain cells react to each hormone. These target cells react because they have receptors for that particular hormone. It's as if the hormone sends out radio signals, and only those cells "tuned in" to that hormone can receive its signal. Here's an analogy: if one hormone is playing Bach and another is transmitting Christmas songs, only the cells tuned to classical stations will pick up the Bach. Those other hormones will keep circulating until they find cells ready to pick up holiday melodies. Once tuned in, the hormone begins to transmit its chemical instructions to the cell.

Hormones aren't the only factors that affect energy. Living an energetic life means more than just increasing physical activity and stamina; it means being alert and interested, excited and stimulated by life and its possibilities. It means recapturing that feeling of being alive that we all have when we are very young and young at heart. The reason that we are able to have those feelings of pleasure and vitality is because of our neurotransmitters. Neurotransmitters are brain chemicals that relay signals between neurons (nerve cells) and communicate information throughout the body and the brain. They tell every organ in your body what to do. They keep your heart beating, your lungs breathing, and your digestive system functioning. They're also responsible for your moods, your ability to think clearly, your appetite, and your sleep patterns. When neurotransmitters are at optimal levels, so is your energy level. When they are out of balance, you can become lethargic, depressed, and/or anxious.

At this time, nobody knows exactly how many neurotransmitters there are in the human body, although scientists have identified more than 100 in the human brain alone. We also don't understand exactly how neurotransmitters work. There are many theories, but the exact mechanisms are still unknown. That means we don't fully understand how medications, foods, or environmental exposure may affect these chemical messengers.

However, we do know that there are two kinds of neurotransmitters: inhibitory and excitatory. An inhibitory neurotransmitter such as serotonin decreases the electrochemical activity of neurons; excitatory neurotransmitters such as dopamine, adrenaline, and endorphins increase electrochemical activity. One is an "on" energy switch, the other is a dimmer. Inhibitory neurotransmitters help create emotional balance and calm the mood. Excitatory neurotransmitters stimulate the brain and raise energy levels.

The consequence of imbalanced hormones and/or neurotransmitters is often depression, and depression leads to lack of energy. If you are suffering from fatigue, you may now want to ask yourself, "Are my hormones in balance? Are my neurotransmitters evened out? If not, why not?" You may want to be tested to find out what, if any, deficiencies are affecting your energy levels (see Chapter 9 for testing options). But you may also want to make some simple lifestyle changes, such as the ones you'll find throughout this book, that can help you regain lost vitality.

Blame It on Your Neurotransmitters

Most of us have experienced neurotransmitter imbalances without even knowing it. Think about times when you have been inexplicably tired, depressed, or moody; situations where you found yourself craving unhealthy foods or were suddenly unable to concentrate. If you don't understand why you're experiencing these things, it just might be that your neurotransmitters are out of whack. In fact, scientists have estimated that as many as 86 percent of Americans may experience depleted neurotransmitter levels, which can be caused by stress, environmental toxins, genetic predisposition, aging, hormonal imbalances, prescription and recreational drug use, poor diet, and alcohol and caffeine intake.

Don't Let Your Life Get Out of Control

Over the years, I have had my own battles with fatigue. Many people have asked me, "How do you do it all? How can you be a wife and a mother and a doctor and write a book, be on TV, and have time to stay in shape?" I believe that I can do all these things because I have learned to compartmentalize my life. I am not all of those things all of the time. There is a time and a place for everything in my life. Yes, you have to be flexible. You have to be adaptable. But you also have to be able to identify your own needs and your own space. You can't let other people influence you to do things you don't want to do or don't have time to do. When you set up those boundaries, it's quite empowering, and empowerment usually translates into energy.

I look at my day and figure out all its elements. I know that I'm going to exercise during this time slot, I'm going to be at my office during these hours, I'm spending these hours with my daughters, we'll have dinner at this time, and my husband and I will spend time together in the evening. This may seem a little militaristic, but I am, of course, flexible (I have to shuffle schedules around at times, but I try to keep to routines as much as possible). There's still plenty of time in the day for unexpected surprises, and I am free to enjoy them because I know my basic schedule and my mind isn't cluttered with "when am I going to fit this in" and "how am I going to get this done." It takes an immense amount of pressure off my shoulders.

If I'm spending my allotted time helping my kids with their schoolwork, I don't take any social calls during my time with my family. You have to make time for the important things, and you have to set priorities. My daughters always know that they're more important than anything else in the world. I won't allow my children to have any memories of their mother on the phone or working in lieu of spending *their* time with *them*. So if it's 7:00 P.M. and the girls are upstairs and calling down "Mommy, Mommy" because they want me to come watch them dance in their bedroom, I don't have to feel guilty if I say no because it's my time to be with my husband and I've already spent the last three hours with them.

What I'm really saying is don't let yourself get distracted or overwhelmed by outside forces. There's a time and a place in my life to get everything done, to do what I have to do for my own body and for my own emotional wellness. Obviously, stressful situations arise. Some people have more stress than others, and in Chapter 4 you'll discover what happens when stress occurs. But if you have a strong body that is made of hormonal balance, exercise, good food, and loving relationships, then you will be able to cope with those unexpected stressors that happen to everyone.

Don't Accept Less Than You Deserve

It's been said that the best lifestyle is one of moderation. But how do you define "moderation"? A friend once told me that everyone needs to set their own level of moderation; that each person has to answer what moderation means for him or herself. I don't agree, because too many people use "moderation" as an excuse not to do their best.

Should a 300-pound woman say her moderation is eating three pizzas by herself at night when she used to eat five? Does the alcoholic set his standard to drink five shots of whisky instead of ten? Should the Vicodin addict be pleased when she takes only 7 pills daily instead of 15?

I don't believe that these are the kinds of standards we should be setting for ourselves. I do believe in taking small steps to achieve large goals, but we cannot live an energized life by settling for small achievements. Life is just too precious. When I was younger, if something depressing or anxiety-producing or tragic happened, I would say, please, just let this day be over. I don't say that anymore because each day that is over is one day lost out of my life. Each day is valuable and I am thankful for it. I recently heard someone say, "When asked what's the best experience of your life, the answer should always be 'the one I am about to have.'" It's never too late to revitalize your life. This book is about helping you obtain maximum energy in your life. If you make the most of the eight essential steps that are in this book and make some positive lifestyle changes, you will feel better, you will look better, you will be better, and you will never again wish for a day to be over.

The Eight Essential Steps

One of the things I love about medicine is that every day is different. Every patient is unique. I never know who is going to walk through the door or what problems they are going to be hoping I can solve. Although every patient I treat is a unique individual, I have found over the years that there are many common complaints, such as weight gain, digestive problems, sleep issues, loss of libido, PMS, and hot flashes, to name a few. There are also many areas of confusion, such as what we should be eating and when, how much sleep we need, how much sexual activity is "normal" as we get older, and most important, why we get so tired. In the following chapters, you'll find the eight factors that address these complaints and clear up their confusions. These eight factors are essential to revitalizing your life and reenergizing your body.

Each chapter is designed to help you understand why that particular step is essential to balancing your hormones as well as to revving up your energy production, how things can go awry, and what you can do to repair and restore your body's vital functions to optimal levels.

If you choose, you can leap right into an action plan, as Chapters 2 through 8 end with a section called "Jump-Start Tips." The Jump Starters are easy steps that don't require a lot of preparation or equipment. You may be surprised at what an energy-packed difference they make.

In the end, it's all about choice. Some choices you make can get you into trouble (hormonally speaking), and others can get you out again. I'm giving you options and challenging you to take the path that will lead you back to health. I've tried to make it as easy for you as I possibly could. Now it's up to you!

CHAPTER 2

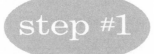

Feed Your
Energy Furnace

My travels in Australia a few years ago put me in contact with some Aborigines, who allowed me to join them on their journey into the desert. Each of them brought along a beetle inside a raw potato. The potato would be sliced in half, with space carved out in the center so that the beetle would have room to mature.

In this way the insect survives and grows. If, in an emergency, the Aborigine can't find food or water in the wilderness, he has a nourishing protein and a source of liquid from this insect.

Imagine being out in the desert for two weeks with nothing but your skill and a potato with an insect inside of it for emergencies (they don't eat the potato, only the insect). It gives them the protein and liquid they need to survive.

This is what I call planning ahead. An excuse I hear all the time is that people don't have the time to prepare what they will eat. They get tied up at work, are running late for their children, or are at an event where they can't be choosy about their meals. The Aborigines taught me that you must always be prepared and have what you need for survival, which in the end is really what life is about. If we treated every meal as if it were a matter of life and death (which it actually is, even if it is not as much of an immediate threat as being caught in the desert), we would surely make time for meal preparation as well as make better, healthier choices. Why is it that when people around the world think of American cuisine it consists of Kentucky Fried Chicken and McDonald's? Fast pace and no pleasure. I've heard that being said about our culture not only as it relates to food, but as it relates to life. We should remember that for humans, as for all other animals, survival is the strongest instinct. Mating is second, and all else is simply icing on the cake. Yet many of us have evolved into eating the cake as being our first priority.

We all know that food gives us energy; it gives us life. Our brains can't function without food, our muscles can't push us forward, our gastrointestinal system can't get rid of toxins, our hearts can't beat, and our glands can't manufacture the hormones that drive our metabolism. Simply put, food is fuel. The more potent the fuel you put into your body, the better the quality of the energy it produces.

There are specific foods that are good for energy, and there are foods you definitely want to avoid. Read on, and you'll find out which is which. Everything we talk about in this chapter is either an energy booster or an energy drainer. Obviously, you want to stay with the energy boosters as much as possible. Here are a few nuggets for how the program will be structured: this is a protein-based food plan, meaning that protein is included in every meal. Carbohydrates are limited, but not eliminated. Fats are divided into good for you and bad for you, but are not eliminated. The goal is to keep your hormone production on a steady keel, and that is accomplished by what you eat, what you eat it with, and when you eat it. (To make your food choices easier, I've designed "Dr. Eva's Energy/Fuel Matrix," 14-days' worth of meal plans and recipes, which you will find in Appendix I at the back of the book.)

FOOD AS YOUR DRUG OF CHOICE

If you've ever had to take a drug for any kind of pain or illness, you probably know about drug interactions—there are warnings on both prescription and over-the-counter medicine labels that caution us against taking certain types of drugs with certain other types of drugs. Some drugs are dangerous when taken with alcohol. Some drugs are less effective when taken with certain foods—for instance, the combination of cholesterol-blocking drugs called statins with grapefruit or grapefruit juice. Chemicals in the grapefruit interact to inhibit certain enzymes from breaking down the statins into more useable compounds in the body. If the statins aren't broken down, they can accumulate in unhealthy amounts, which can cause muscle and liver damage.

On the other hand, grapefruit with all its enzymes actually speeds up metabolism in a positive way. If you are not on statins, I encourage its use on a daily basis. (This is not to be confused with the grapefruit diet fad that requires people eat grapefruit all day, with a few very small meals to go along with it. People who tried this diet lost weight, but they also got sick because they were not taking in enough nutrients. Any fad diet is a bad diet.) When I was a little girl, my Eastern European parents used to make me eat half a grapefruit before every meal. My American friends thought this was a bizarre custom. Hard as I tried to rebel against this ritual, my parents were unrelenting. I was the odd kid who ate grapefruit all the time. I am now grateful for this bit of "insanity," since the research on grapefruit is irrefutable, and I owe at least part of my fast metabolic rate to this ritual.

On a similar note, I had friends growing up whose parents would insist on giving them cod liver oil daily. Not only did my peers and I think their parents were crazy, but the cod liver oil also had a horrible flavor. We now know that cod liver oil is very good for you and contains omega-3 fatty acids, vitamin A, and vitamin D. There is something to be said about folklore and old wives' tales as they relate to food—it's part of what I mean by learning from the past. Even though I may utilize some of the most cutting-edge science and technology for my patients, I never discount information just because it seems "old school" or is based on ancient tradition.

We no longer rely solely on old wives' tales to let us know what we should be eating. Until recently, most of us never thought about putting the words *science* and *food* together. But scientists are now helping us to understand the chemical aspects of food and how those chemicals interact with the chemicals in our systems.

Probably the best advice I can give my patients is something that was first said by the ancient Greek physician Hippocrates: "Let food be thy medicine and medicine be thy food." Every bite of food we take, from the first one in the morning to last snack at night, has a direct, chemical-based effect on us. Your choices can make a difference in how you feel and how you look, how you function in the world, and how much energy you will have to get you through the day.

The problem is that much of what we eat today—the huge amounts of sugar and processed carbohydrates (which we will get to shortly)—does not react well with our bodies' chemistry. Sugar and carbs specifically affect hormones, and two hormones in particular affect our energy levels: insulin and cortisol.

❖ **The Insulin Factor:** Insulin is one of the body's key hormones. It works with a partner, glucagon, to regulate how the body utilizes food for fuel and therefore energy. Insulin is a hormone designed to take excess glucose (sugar) from dietary carbohydrates and store it. Not only does it store glucose, but it also locks it up so it can't be released easily.Glucagon, insulin's biological opposite, mobilizes stored energy (primarily carbohydrates), to be circulated in the bloodstream as a source of energy. Its primary job is to release stored carbohydrate, in the form of glucose, from the liver so that it can be used for energy. So . . .

Insulin = Stored energy
Glucagon = Released energy

An imbalance between these two hormones is usually seen as elevated insulin levels. Excess blood sugar usually responds to elevated insulin by dropping down dramatically, which will decimate your energy level and give you that well-known "sugar crash." Or it can respond by staying elevated, in which case the body's cells can't handle the excess and simply don't allow any more sugar or insulin to come in. This is known as insulin resistance, which is the body's inability to respond to and use the insulin it produces. This can eventually lead to a variety of conditions, including the accumulation of body fat, diabetes, heart disease, and a decrease in energy levels. So . . .

Excess blood sugar = insulin resistance

❖ **The Cortisol Factor:** Cortisol is a hormone produced in the adrenal glands that is critical to your body's ability to mediate stress. This came in very handy in the age of the caveman; cortisol is part of the fight-or-flight process that prepares you to either face and hopefully vanquish your enemy or run away as fast as your feet can take you. Today's stressors may not be as dramatic as facing a hungry saber-toothed tiger, but they are quite a bit more varied. Stressors can be physical, biological, environmental, or even social, from a weekend warrior's overexertion to a sudden viral infection to a chronically abusive screaming boss. Cortisol helps you cope and allows you to respond to different stressors in different ways. However, long-term exposure to unremitting stress (taking care of a parent or child with a chronic illness; a chaotic lifestyle that never slows down) will have dire consequences for your health, as too much cortisol can produce extensive biological damage and is a leading cause of premature aging and fatigue.

Cortisol has many actions in the body, and one ultimate goal of cortisol secretion is the provision of energy for the body. Cortisol stimulates fat and carbohydrate metabolism for fast energy. It also stimulates insulin release and maintenance of blood sugar levels. The end result of these actions is an increase in appetite. That's why chronic or poorly managed stress may lead you to eat too much, which can show up as weight gain or difficulty losing unwanted pounds. So . . .

Excess cortisol = premature aging and fatigue

As you read the rest of this chapter, you'll discover why these two hormones are so enmeshed with what you eat. You'll also learn that when you eat can be just as important as what you put in your mouth.

Wait . . . You're Eating *Again?*

Karen is in her mid-40's. She has always been thin and active. She jogged three hours daily for many years. She was recently divorced; although she and her husband had frequent sex and didn't use birth control, they never had any children. In retrospect she probably didn't have enough body fat on her to get pregnant (that's another story). She scheduled her appointment with me because she no longer had the energy to do *anything:* not to jog, not to go out on dates, not even to get to work on time, since she simply couldn't get out of bed in the morning. During the three years that it took for her divorce to be finalized, she reacted to her stress by not eating. She had no appetite in the morning, so she didn't eat breakfast, and since she was always late for work, her boss agreed to let her come in late as long as she worked through lunch. She was usually so busy at work that she'd forget to order food and would then decide to pick something up on her way home so she could eat in bed while watching TV. She did try to eat a healthy dinner by getting a salad and chicken or fish, as well as a fruit desert. But by the time she got home after not eating all day, she was hypoglycemic—in other words, her blood sugar had bottomed out, creating extreme fatigue. So she'd stick her healthy meal in the fridge for another day, make herself a Hungry Man frozen dinner, and enjoy the company of Ben and Jerry for dessert.

Most of us have been taught the rule of three when it comes to eating. Three meals a day—breakfast, lunch, and dinner—with perhaps an occasional snack before bedtime. That's the way it's supposed to be, isn't it? After all, we've been doing it all our lives. Turns out, it may not be the best thing for us after all.

In fact, we should be eating every three to four hours. This doesn't mean a full meal every time; it includes small in-between-meal snacks such as a handful of almonds, some cashews and raisins, a piece of string cheese, a couple of scoops of cottage cheese, even a small piece of beef jerky (this will last a long time in a purse or pocket—a trick I learned while skiing for hours far away from any kind of food source). Going longer than that between meals or snacks will lower blood sugar levels. Low blood sugar levels equal low energy levels. Low blood sugar levels trigger the pituitary gland to release adrenocorticotropic hormone (ACTH) which in turn raises cortisol levels, which in turn causes blood sugar levels to rise. When that happens, your hormones are not balanced. What you end up with is radical swings in blood sugar, a constant cycle of adrenal stress, and a roller-coaster ride of high energy and bottoming out.

Here's what happens when you go too long between meals (we're using "meals" in the generic sense of "having something to eat," which includes full breakfasts, lunches, dinners, and light snacks). Suppose you are on a hiking trip and your backpack full of food and supplies goes over the side of the mountain (luckily you don't go with it). You're now hiking for hours with nothing to eat. You come upon a lake and nearby you discover a nest containing eight duck eggs. Food! You're so hungry, you're tempted to eat all the eggs at once, but you realize that you're better off eating one every few hours to spread out your energy resources. And you're right. If you eat eight eggs at once, you'll consume more calories than your body will be able to use.

The same thing happens when you eat three large meals a day with many hours of noneating in between. Suppose you eat lunch at noon. Between getting out of work, fighting traffic to get home, taking the kids to soccer practice, and then finally finding time to prepare and cook your next meal, it could be seven or eight o'clock before you eat dinner. By that time not only are you exhausted, but you will also usually eat more than you need because you're so hungry.

And of course, we all know "a friend" (okay—we've done it ourselves) who has gone on a starvation diet, eating nothing but a few carrot sticks and celery stalks in the hope of losing weight (there will be more about weight loss later in this chapter). We know this can't last, and when we can't hold out any longer, we end up binge-eating.

Not too long ago, I had a patient named Hilary who came into my office for the first time. When I asked her to fill out some information forms, I could see her hands were shaking. This concerned me, as it could be a symptom of any number of serious ailments. When I asked her about it, she said, "Oh, this happens all the time when I get hungry." Then she told me that since she was trying to lose weight, she had had a diet shake for breakfast at about 8:00 A.M. and had skipped lunch altogether. It was now about 3:00 P.M. She did confess that when she got home, she would more than likely eat too much for dinner, including dessert, but that it would "balance out the lack of calories" she had consumed all day. She also said this was a pattern for her, and was probably why she had such difficulty losing weight.

I get patients like Hilary in my office all the time who have told me of their starving/bingeing habits. What happens then is that the hypothalamus (a part of the brain located just above the brain stem that links the nervous system with the endocrine system) gets very confused. One of its primary functions is to maintain the body's metabolism and energy status quo. It senses the nutrients that are circulating around the body and adjusts the body's metabolism to try and make the most efficient use of those nutrients. A pattern of starving and bingeing negatively affects the hypothalamus's ability to sense these nutrients. To get your metabolism working efficiently again, you basically have to "retrain" the hypothalamus. So . . .

Waiting too long between meals = inefficient metabolism
and an energy roller coaster

Eating every four hours = efficient metabolism
and steady energy production

I was able to convince both Karen and Hilary that they needed to be on a schedule of having meals and snacks every three to four hours. They both complied, and both report that they have more than enough energy to get through the work day, take part in some nighttime activities, and enjoy their lives once again.

THE ENERGY INFLUENCERS: NUTRIENTS

To create energy of any kind, you need a source of fuel. To create heat, for instance, you need to burn fuel—twigs or logs or coal or other flammable substances. Human beings also need to burn fuel to create energy, and in a process called metabolism, the fuel that we burn is food—more specifically, the nutrients we get from the food we eat. There are three principle types of nutrients used as energy sources by the body:

- ❖ Proteins
- ❖ Carbohydrates
- ❖ Fats

The food you eat is broken down into its basic nutrient components in your digestive system. Those nutrients pass through the liver or circulate in the bloodstream until they find a cell that needs fuel. They then move into the microscopic energy factories called mitochondria, which are found in every cell in your body (except for red blood cells). There are many millions of mitochondria in our bodies, and each one needs to be supplied with the proper nutrients to keep running efficiently.

The actual process of converting food into energy is known as respiration, and it is how cells get energy from sugars. Energy is stored in glucose molecules, which are released into the bloodstream where they can be converted immediately to energy in the cells when needed. It's like having an energy bank account. We put energy into a savings account until it's needed, and then we make a withdrawal when necessary.

This process involves a complex series of biochemical reactions (known as the Krebs cycle) that eventually converts fats, proteins, and carbohydrates into a molecule called adenosine triphosphate, or ATP. ATP is vital to our survival. It supplies energy needed to contract muscles, including skeletal and heart muscles; allows chromosomes to function; enables electric messages to be sent along your nerve cells; and acts as an "on-off" switch to a host of vital chemical reactions in the body.

The conversion of nutrients to ATP is an aerobic process, meaning that it requires oxygen, which is why exercise (which increases oxygenation) is good for you. But it also requires the presence of many other vitamins, minerals, and amino acids, including vitamins B_1, B_2, B_3, and C, iron, magnesium, manganese, and phosphorus, arginine, cysteine, glutamine, carnitine, and tyrosine—just to name a few. That's why it's so important that your diet be nutritionally sound (and that's why Step #1 is Feeding Your Energy Furnace). Your energy production depends on it.

In other words, metabolism works by combining the oxygen we breathe and the nutrients we eat and turning them into energy, the fuel for life.

When there are nutritional deficiencies, energy production is inefficient, and the body begins to experience the dreaded "F" word . . . fatigue. When all the necessary nutrients are present, energy production will be smooth and efficient.

THE THREE ENERGY NUTRIENTS: PROTEINS, CARBS, AND FATS

Now that you know how the inclusive category of "food" influences the way your body works, it's time to talk about specific foods and food groups, and why so many of them are so good for us and our energy production—and so bad for us when they're overconsumed. You'll learn about why cutting out carbohydrates altogether (as some diet advocates suggest) can be devastating for your health and energy production—and why eating too many of the wrong kind can be just as bad. You'll find out about the pros and cons of wheat, dairy, proteins, and fats (you may be surprised to learn that fats are essential for a body's health).

We are incredibly lucky to live in a country where there is such a wide variety of foods from which to choose. When I was traveling through Kazakhstan and Tibet, I loved the food because it was always fresh and organic. However, there was no variety. You could travel from one region to the next and there was very little difference in the food that was being offered and the way it was being prepared. People ate the same thing for breakfast as they ate for lunch and dinner. In many places, they are most concerned about getting anything at all to eat and don't really care that it's the same thing they've eaten for most of their lives. In the States, we have the luxury of getting bored eating the same things over and over. I suggest you to take advantage of the variety available to you and appreciate what it can do for your health and well-being.

Once you understand how different foods work in your body, you'll begin to look at food in a different way. You'll want to make changes for yourself and for your family. You'll begin to introduce yourself to foods that may be new to your palate but that can contribute to a rich and complex diet. Not so many years ago, you had to travel to several different ethnic markets or specialty shops to find anything other than a "meat and potatoes" menu. Now, virtually every supermarket offers a huge variety of organic and ethnic foods. I urge you to try foods that may be unfamiliar to you. You may not like everything you try. But you will surely find something you enjoy, and then you can add it into your food repertoire, one bite at a time.

Proteins, fats, and carbohydrates are also known as macronutrients. The body gets its energy from the breakdown of these foods into nutrients such as glucose (from carbs), amino acids (from proteins), and fatty acids (from fats). It takes all three macronutrients to keep energy levels at their best. Proteins are high priority, followed by fats and carbs. Pasta with meat sauce is better for you than plain pasta or pasta with tomato sauce. A meal that consists only of broccoli and brown rice sprinkled with soy sauce may contain vitamins, but it will also throw off your hormonal balance. Since this meal has no protein or fat, it is a pure "carb load" and may cause oversecretion of insulin by the pancreas. That can cause the pancreas to crash and your cortisol to flatline. This type of meal will not provide you with the energy you need. Later in this chapter, I will explain the role of each food group in energy production and show you how to mix and match to get the biggest bang for your energy buck.

PROTEINS AND ENERGY

Here is the number one edict of the Fatigue Solution program: eat protein at every meal. If you want energy all day, eat protein all day. I'm not saying don't eat carbs or fats as well, but I am saying that you should look for a protein first and then combine it with other nutrients.

From Dr. Eva's Files

Sarah, a 40-year-old mother of two toddlers, came to me because she was "crashing" every afternoon and barely had enough stamina to make it through until her kids were in bed. She couldn't understand this, she said, because she had taken my advice and had started eating breakfast every morning, something she never used to do. I asked her to describe a typical morning meal. She proudly told me she had a banana every day sprinkled with wheat germ, and a glass of orange juice. "Where is the protein?" I asked. "For breakfast?" she said, looking confused. "For every meal," I told her. "But," she said, "I love having fruit for breakfast. I don't want to give it up." "You don't have to. Just don't have it every day. And when you do have it, add one scoop of vanilla whey-based protein powder into your juice or just drink a glass of whole milk and you won't believe the difference it makes." A few weeks later, she returned to the office and was excited to inform me that she was feeling much better and was now able to get through a day and actually have fun with her children. Best of all, she and her husband now share a leisurely Sunday breakfast of two-egg omelets with green peppers, tomatoes, goat cheese, onions, and spices. Great moments and great memories—and the energy to enjoy it all.

For one thing, protein works well with the appetite control centers in your brain that tell you when you've had enough to eat (much better than carbohydrates do). Proteins release enzymes in the stomach that make you feel full. This is related to peptides (certain amino acids) called cholecystokinin (CCK) and peptide YY that turn on satiety signals. That means when you eat protein, you release CCK and peptide YY, and you are going to be much less likely to overeat. And, when you eat a meal that has a greater ratio of proteins to carbs, your blood sugar stabilizes and your insulin response improves.

Protein also increases your basal metabolic rate (BMR), which is the number of calories your body burns at rest to maintain body functions. The more calories your body burns, the higher your energy level.

Proteins are the fundamental components of all living cells. That pretty much says it all. Every part and system of the body needs proteins to function. In addition to building, repairing, and replacing tissue, protein helps to stabilize blood sugar, enabling us to burn more sugar between meals.

The easiest way to determine what foods are proteins is to remember that if it crawls, walks, or swims, it's a protein. Unlike fats and carbohydrates, there are no unhealthy proteins. If you eat more protein than is necessary (we'll get to adequate amounts later), the excess is eliminated through the kidneys. The body doesn't store protein the way it stores fat.

The best foods to eat for protein are not necessarily those that are highest in grams of protein, but those that are highest in quality. In general, animal proteins are considered highly digestible and higher quality than plant sources of protein, in part because plant sources also have a lot more fiber, which is indigestible. The problem with plant protein is that you have to eat a tremendous amount of it to get the same amount of protein as you'd find in a small serving of chicken or steak, for instance.

Here are some tips about choosing quality proteins:

- ❖ **Don't be afraid of red meat:** Red meat has tons of vitamin B, especially B_{12} (required for normal gene function, energy production, and the formation of blood cells), that other foods such as fish and chicken don't have. Vegetarians, especially, have to be extra careful that they are getting enough of the B vitamins in their diets because the Bs are the most important vitamins in terms of energy production. B_1 (thiamin) is necessary for adrenal gland function, proper immune performance, and the synthesis of neurotransmitters. B_2 (riboflavin) is required for energy production and oxygen utilization. B_3 and B_5 are also necessary for energy production. Some of my patients tell me they don't want to eat red meat because of the cholesterol or because of the hormones that cattle ingest, but if you buy lean organic beef, you won't have those concerns.

Choose the leanest cuts of meat you can find. Look for the words *loin* or *round* in the name. If you're buying ground beef, look for ground sirloin or ground round, and choose packages labeled *lean* or *extra lean.* Of course, these cuts of meat, especially if you're buying organic, are the most expensive. So buy the best cut of meat you can afford.

❖ **For variety, try chicken and turkey.** Chicken and turkey are healthy sources of the amino acid tyrosine, which boosts levels of dopamine and norepinephrine, brain chemicals that can help you feel more alert and focused. Don't forget that there are many ways to serve poultry. You can get lean ground chicken and ground turkey for healthy alternative-style burgers, meat loaf, or meat sauce. Chicken and turkey can also be used in chili, tacos, and most other dishes that are traditionally made with ground beef. To make chicken and turkey even healthier, cut off the excess fat and remove the skin.

❖ **Eat fish, but don't go overboard.** Fish is a naturally lean source of protein. Seafood is especially good because of the omega-3 fatty acids that are found in it. There are some concerns about eating fish, however, because of the issue of mercury overload, which is why the U.S. Food and Drug Administration (FDA) recommends that you avoid large predatory fish, including shark, swordfish, king mackerel, and tilefish, which contain the highest levels of mercury.

❖ **Beans, beans, beans.** Many beans are a wonderful source of protein and are especially critical for those choosing a vegetarian diet (plus they're loaded with valuable fiber). Lentils are a particularly good choice because one cup has 17 grams of protein with only .75 grams of fat. A two-ounce extra-lean sirloin steak has the same amount of protein but six times the fat. Some other healthy beans include black beans, chickpeas, kidney beans, garbanzo beans, and legumes, to name a few. If you're cooking with dried beans, it's best to soak them overnight before preparing them in any dish because beans can cause digestive problems. The good news is that there are several products on the market that can help prevent gas before it starts.

❖ **Discover quinoa.** Quinoa (*kee-nwa*), a South American grain that has a slightly nutty flavor, is one of the few complete plant proteins. Although it is usually categorized as a grain, technically it is a seed that is rich in essential fats, vitamins, and minerals and an excellent source of calcium, iron, and vitamins B and E. More and more of my patients are coming and telling me about this particular protein. I had never heard of it until a couple of years ago. The first few times patients told me about it, I was actually embarrassed to ask what it was, so don't feel bad if you've never heard of it—just give it a try. You cook quinoa much as you cook rice: bring two cups of water to a boil with one cup of quinoa; cover at a low simmer and cook for 14–18 minutes or until the germ separates from the seed. The cooked germ looks like a tiny curl and should have a slight bite to it (like al dente pasta).

❖ **Go nuts.** Nuts are loaded with protein, fiber, and minerals, all great sources of energy. Nuts also contain coenzyme Q10 (CoQ10), a nutrient that helps our cells produce energy. They're also a good source of omega-3 fatty acids, a type of unsaturated fats which provides energy to the muscles and organs. Many nuts also contain magnesium, a mineral that plays a vital role in converting sugar into energy. Research suggests magnesium deficiency can drain your energy (magnesium is also found in whole grains, particularly bran cereals, and in some types of fish, including halibut). The best nuts for snacking and to use as condiments are walnuts, pecans, macadamias, pine nuts, hazelnuts, cashews, and almonds. Keeping some on hand will give you a tasty and effective alternative to unhealthy snacks such as candy bars or potato chips. Even better, roast them a bit to add flavor and make their nutrients more bioavailable.

The whole idea is to eat as much of a variety of proteins as possible. If you eat only one protein source, you limit the number of amino acids you will consume. If you want to get optimum performance from your body and optimum energy output, you need to be exposed to a complete pool of amino acids on a regular basis.

The Incredible Edible Egg

Eggs are rich in nutrients, in amino acids and key vitamins and minerals. Egg whites are almost pure protein. And egg whites contain an enzyme that negates the yolk of the egg, so you're not going to get an increase of cholesterol. Many people have given up eating whole eggs due to fear of cholesterol. Eggs do have a lot of cholesterol; however, only a small amount of the cholesterol in food passes into the blood. Saturated and trans fats (see page 41) actually do much more damage as far as cholesterol is concerned. Studies have shown that the cholesterol in eggs does raise the cholesterol in the body, but it raises the HDL (good) cholesterol that gets elevated by the eggs. That's why the total cholesterol goes up—but HDL is actually a cardio-protective cholesterol. There's no reason to be concerned about a somewhat elevated cholesterol if the elevation is in HDL.

Whole eggs contain a plethora of energy-producing nutrients. Yolks contain choline (a member of the vitamin B family), necessary for the synthesis of acetylcholine, one of the major neurotransmitters in the body essential for brain health and cognitive efficiency. Eggs are an energy superfood. In the Fatigue Solution program, you can eat up to six whole eggs a week. Consult your physician regarding your specific number of eggs. If you have cholesterol or heart problems, your health professional may recommend fewer whole eggs.

Do you need to buy organic eggs? There is disagreement on this issue. Some studies have found that organic eggs have, on average, one-third less cholesterol than commercial eggs. They also have four to six times the vitamin D, a quarter less saturated fat, twice the omega-3 fatty acid, and three times the vitamin E. However, a 2010 study conducted by the United States Department of Agriculture (USDA) found that there is virtually no difference. USDA scientists measured the amount of thick albumen (part of the egg white) in a variety of eggs. The greater amount of thick albumen, the more nutritious the egg. And they found no differences between organic and nonorganic eggs. So if organic eggs are out of your price range or are not available in your area, don't worry. Just enjoy your eggs scrambled, poached, soft- or hard-boiled, or even better, as your favorite omelet cooked up with fresh herbs and green vegetables such as spinach or asparagus.

Remember that eggs should always be cooked thoroughly. Raw eggs are breeding places for salmonella (a dangerous and deadly bacteria). Federal researchers estimate that more than 130,000 people are sickened every year and 30 die as a result of contaminated eggs.

CARBOHYDRATES AND ENERGY

Decades ago, when I was on the ski team in high school, we used to get "instant energy" by chugging from a jar of honey right before we'd go out to compete. It was instant energy all right—it gave you an immediate rush that was gone in an instant. What I've learned since then is that you can't rely on the instant energy you get from carbohydrates to help you perform for the rest of the day.

What are carbohydrates anyway? They are mainly sugars and starches and are one of the three principle types of nutrients used as energy sources by the body. Carbohydrates are made up of chains of sugar molecules. Even carbs that don't seem to be sugary—such as bread, bagels, and pasta—are made up of sugar molecules.

Carbs supply energy to every cell in your body by turning the carbohydrate to glucose (sugar). The body uses as much glucose as it needs for immediate fuel; the unused portion is converted to glycogen and stored in your liver and muscle cells. If there is any glucose left over, it is turned to fat. If you need a quick charge of energy for, say, catching a bus, escaping from a burning building, or any kind of emergency situation, the body will release stores of glycogen. If you need energy for a longer period of time, such as playing a nine-inning baseball game or taking a long hike on a mountain trail, the body turns to fat for fuel.

One of the problems we have in the modern age is that many of us seem to be in a constant state of stress. That's what happened to 25-year-old Phoebe, who came to see me after she had gained 20 pounds over six months. "I don't understand how this happened," she said. "Especially because lately I've been living on a couple cans of soda and some crackers and cheese." When I asked why she was doing that, Phoebe explained that she never eats when she's stressed and that her stress level had recently skyrocketed. It seemed she had just been given new responsibilities at work, and she was having a hard time coping with the new technologies she had to learn. On top of that, her mother had been diagnosed with Alzheimer's, and her son had just announced that he had dropped out of college and was coming home to live with her. Adding to all of this, Phoebe now found that with this "inexplicable" weight gain, none of her clothes fit her anymore and she had nothing to wear to work. So she ended up spending her newly increased paycheck for a new wardrobe, and she was none the better for it.

Whether it's a job, a relationship, being part of the "sandwich generation," or having too many demands on us and too little time (which all women can relate to), our adrenals are working overtime. This leads to a constant state of excess cortisol production, which stimulates glucose production. This excess glucose ends up as stored fat in the body.

When adrenaline runs through our bodies, it signals cells to release fat for energy. But when there is too much adrenaline (due to the constant stress), the cells become unresponsive to these signals. At the same time, the high levels of cortisol are producing increased fat storage, which leads to obesity, which leads insulin resistance, metabolic syndrome, diabetes, heart disease, and fatigue.

But too much stress isn't the only factor that can lead to these hormonal imbalances. Another contributing factor is the overconsumption of simple carbohydrates. When you eat a sweet snack and gulp down a soda, for example, you're loading your body with sugar, which triggers an influx of insulin to prevent excess blood sugar. This influx of insulin can in turn cause a dramatic drop in blood sugar a few hours later, meaning your energy runs out and you experience that sugar crash. The body, sensing a problem with low blood sugar and reduced energy, produces a surge of adrenal stress hormones, including adrenaline and cortisol, and a vicious cycle begins.

Contrary to some popular diet plans, we need to include some carbohydrates in our daily fare. We can live without carbs, but not well. What you need to know is that not all carbs are bad for you, and eliminating one entire food group is not the best thing you can do for your body. Carbs provide us with fiber, antioxidants, and brain fuel, and they raise serotonin levels, which makes us feel less depressed and more energized. On the other hand, they do raise insulin levels. Too much insulin and your blood-sugar level plummets, dragging your energy down with it. You also have to concern yourself with developing diabetes from too much sugar. Once you've got diabetes, that's an entirely different matter.

Some carbs also provide us with fiber, important to the digestive process because it gets food to move more quickly through the large intestine, reducing the risk of digestive disorders, including constipation, which is commonly caused by low fiber intake. Fiber also helps us feel full after a meal, which can help keep us from overeating and reduce our tendencies to clamor for snacks before bedtime.

Carbohydrates rich in fiber include green, leafy vegetables such as spinach, watercress, lettuce, and a wide variety of sprouts. Add in vegetables such as tomatoes, carrots, pea pods, asparagus, zucchini, peppers, radishes, and cucumbers; and cooked cruciferous vegetables such as broccoli, kale, cauliflower, cabbage, and Brussels sprouts, and your fiber intake will be more than adequate.

Fruits and vegetables are among the best sources of carbohydrates you can eat. Try to include fruits that are rich in natural antioxidants (chemical substances that help protect against cell damage) and vitamin C. Blueberries and strawberries, for instance, are rich in antioxidants, and they have anti-inflammatory and blood-thinning effects as well.

All fruits and vegetables are good for you, whether they are fresh, frozen, dried, or canned (when choosing canned fruit, look for labels that say *no sugar added*). They can be eaten raw, steamed, roasted, boiled, sautéed, microwaved, or stir-fried. The best idea is to have a variety of different types of fruit and vegetables from all the different color groups (yellow, green, and red).

What, No Dessert?

One of the differences Westerners notice when they travel to the Far East or parts of the Middle East is that dessert is not usually part of the culture. They might have fruit for dessert, but there is not much in the way of cookies or cake or chocolate or candies. There are no snack foods such as chips or cheese doodles. In countries such as Afghanistan and Pakistan, they add sweetness to their meals of lamb, veal, or pork by serving grapes, raisins, and dates in bowls on the table, which you are expected to eat during the meal, not after it.

The Controversial Carbs: Corn and Wheat

Two of the most controversial carbs in the American diet are corn and wheat. Neither of these carbs is inherently bad for you. It's the way they're used—or rather, overused—in food production that makes them an unhealthy addition to our diet.

Let's start with corn. Most people think that serving corn is a good vegetable option. You might be surprised to learn, however, that corn is not a vegetable at all—it's a grain. It's still a tantalizing treat for a backyard cookout. But in the past several decades, something has happened to our delicious ear of corn. In two distinct ways, this sweet summer treat has turned into a danger for our society's future.

First, let's talk about high-fructose corn syrup (HFCS), a common sweetener and preservative, made by changing the sugar (glucose) in cornstarch to fructose—another form of sugar. The end product extends the shelf life of processed foods and is cheaper than sugar. And it is now found in an astounding array of foods: candy, beverages, cereals, breads, cookies, crackers, yogurt, ice cream, salad dressing, steak sauce, pancake syrup, pasta sauce, ketchup, canned soups, fruit juice, soft drinks, and even cough syrup. Unfortunately for us, studies have shown that unlike glucose, fructose is readily converted to fat by the liver, leading to an excessive concentration of fats and lipoproteins (compounds of protein that carry fats and fatlike substances, such as cholesterol, in the blood) in the body. This can eventually lead to plaque buildup in the blood vessels, gout, kidney stones, obesity, and type 2 diabetes, all of which put a strain on our energy production.

The second problem with corn has to do with cows (and chickens, too) and the fact that corn has entered every aspect of the food chain. Take beef, for instance. Almost all beef that we eat comes from cattle that are fed primarily corn, corn husks, and corn stalks. Cows are not designed to live on corn; they are designed to live on grasses. However, one of the quickest ways to fatten a cow is to feed it primarily corn. And that's a problem because beef that comes from corn-fed cattle is high in saturated fats, which is known to clog arteries. All that saturated fat, coupled with the antibiotics cattle are fed to keep them from getting sick, is making us sick instead.

What to do? We want to get the vitamin B for energy production that red meat provides, but we don't want the saturated fat and antibiotics. The answer is to go organic if possible. I know that organic beef and chicken can be expensive. Not too long ago, you could only find organic meats at Whole Foods and local health-food stores. These days, however, although most large chain supermarkets carry organic foods at lower prices, you can't find them everywhere. My parents live in a suburb 25 miles outside of New York City. They were visiting me in California, and I was trying to help my mother lose weight (which she did—she lost 30 pounds in 30 days!) and we were concerned that when she went back home she wouldn't be able to find the same kinds of stores we have out here. There is no Whole Foods where she lives. There was only a small organic section in her closest supermarket. She does have a farmer's market near her on the weekends, but it isn't organic. So you may have to make a bit of an effort to find the healthiest foods, but aren't you and your family worth it?

Is Organic Always Necessary?

Not everything you buy needs to be organic. Here are some simple rules on when to buy organic and when it's not necessary:

Buy organic when the skin is thin. Fruits and vegetables with thin skins that are difficult to remove or that you usually eat should be organic. They do not have the same type of barrier against pesticides that thick-skinned fruits and veggies have. Thin skinned examples include apples, strawberries, peaches, raspberries, blueberries, blackberries, grapes, pears, cherries, nectarines, celery, potatoes, and carrots. Thick skinned examples include avocados, bananas, eggplant, corn, kiwi, papaya, mangoes, squash, oranges, and grapefruit.

Leafy greens should be organic. Anything that is leafy such as lettuce should be organic because you can't completely wash every leaf. Vegetables that should be organic include all types of lettuce, kale, spinach, collard greens, mustard greens, and Swiss chard. Vegetables that don't need to be organic include broccoli, cabbage, asparagus, cauliflower, and sweet potatoes.

Dairy should be organic. This industry uses a lot of hormones and antibiotics, so buy organic milk, cheese, and yogurt whenever possible. Also, organic milk has higher levels of omega-3 fatty acids, which is good for your health.

Meat and Poultry should be organic. The caveat about hormones and antibiotics applies here as well.

Fish and seafood do not need to be organic. Fish live in the ocean and (hopefully) do not encounter as many pesticides and toxins as other foods, except for the mercury as explained on page 29.

Controversial Carb #2: Wheat

The second "problem" grain in the American diet is wheat. And once again, wheat in itself is not inherently bad for you—it's the *overconsumption* of wheat that is the issue. Wheat is, in fact, deeply embedded in the food culture of North America and many other regions of the world. Bread, pasta, pizza, bagels, cereal, crackers, cakes, and muffins are just some of the foods made with wheat.

Like corn, wheat in its original state is good for you. It's got dietary fiber, manganese, and magnesium. However, the main nutrients in wheat (not to mention the fiber) come from its hard outer layer, called bran, and the germ, the inner part of a wheat kernel, both of which are removed when the grain is milled to produce white flour.

One of the biggest problems we have with eating so much wheat is gluten, a gluey protein substance occurring in cereal grains such as wheat, rye, barley, and corn. A little gluten won't harm most people. But most people ingest more than a "little" gluten every day. In fact, most of us aren't even aware of how much wheat we eat in a day.

I have a patient named Gloria who came to see me because she was extremely tired—she was sneaking into the ladies' lounge in the department store where she worked to take a quick nap almost every afternoon. She had been gaining weight recently, her stomach was bloated, and she was getting increasingly depressed. Since these are all symptoms of gluten sensitivity, I asked her to describe what she'd eaten the day before her visit to my office. Gloria's first meal of the day was a bowl of cereal for breakfast. Midmorning at work she grabbed some pretzels from the vending machine (better than a candy bar, right?). She had a lunch meeting in the conference room and the boss sent out for pizza for everyone so they didn't have to stop working. Later in the day, Gloria snacked on a crunchy granola bar. Then she'd had late dinner plans with friends at a Chinese restaurant. She'd decided to order something light so she went for cold noodles with sesame sauce and a spring roll. Let's review: wheat for breakfast, wheat for snack, wheat for lunch, a late-day wheat snack, and wheat for dinner. Gluten overload, anyone?

But wait. As if it isn't difficult enough to avoid gluten in your diet, it turns out that gluten is also used as a thickener or stabilizing agent in products such as ice cream, canned soup, pie filling, salad dressing, and ketchup. In fact, if you find any of the following words on food labels, it usually means that a grain containing gluten has been used:

❖ Stabilizer

❖ Modified food starch (prominent in candy)

❖ Monosodium glutamate (MSG)

❖ Flavoring

❖ Emulsifier

❖ Hydrolyzed vegetable protein

❖ Plant protein

❖ Caramel coloring

The human body doesn't really have the capability to digest this much gluten; therefore, gluten causes all sorts of problems and disorders, from ear infections and stomachaches, to the common problems of gas and bloating, constipation, and last but not least, lethargy.

I tested Gloria for gluten sensitivity, but while waiting for the results, I advised Gloria to keep a food log of her diet for a week so she would be more aware of how much wheat she was consuming. Her results came back positive for gluten sensitivity. Then I asked her to cut down on the wheat and add more protein, fruits, and vegetables to her meals. I told her she didn't have to cut out wheat entirely but to be careful that she wasn't eating it all day every day. In two months, when Gloria came for a follow-up visit, she had lost 12 pounds and her symptoms were gone. And, she said, she still had pizza for lunch occasionally and her favorite pasta for dinner—just not on the same day.

The good news is that there are an increasing number of gluten-free products on the market, including gluten-free breads and pastas. But it's important to note that *wheat free* doesn't necessarily mean *gluten free*. The product may still contain rye, barley, or spelt ingredients that contain gluten. And many products that are labeled *gluten free* are higher in sugar, fat, calories, and carbohydrates than similar products that contain gluten.

Tiger and Me

During the course of writing this book I got my first dog ever! One day Tiger (his name) and I were reviewing some doggy commands in the park. I wanted to give him a treat for his good behavior, but all I had on me was a granola bar. *Oh well,* I thought. *He's been a good boy and I need to reward him.* When another dog owner saw me break off a piece of my bar and start to kneel down, she rushed toward me and said, "Don't feed that to him. Dogs can't digest gluten. They don't have the enzymes for this. You'll make him sick." Of course, she was right, and I felt terribly guilty. A little while later, I went over to explain that I was a new dog owner and to excuse myself for my lack of doggy snack etiquette when I saw her pull out chocolate chip cookies and diet sodas for her own personal snack. If a dog's diet is of such concern to its owner, why isn't the owner's diet of more concern? Why should we be more concerned about our pets than ourselves? (For the record, I now give Tiger only food intended for dogs. Live and learn.)

Gluten also causes problems for people who are truly allergic to it and have what is known as celiac disease, a digestive disorder that interferes with the absorption of nutrients from food. Some common symptoms of celiac disease are diarrhea, decreased appetite, stomachache and bloating, poor growth, and weight loss. This is a serious disease that requires strict adherence to a gluten-free diet.

Many more people are not truly allergic to gluten but have gluten sensitivities (as Gloria did). This does not require complete elimination of wheat from the diet. If you have gluten sensitivity, you can consume moderate amounts of wheat and wheat products. But it does take careful monitoring on your part. You may have to experiment to judge exactly how much you can comfortably consume, but eventually you'll find what is right for your body.

Perhaps your doctor tested you for a gluten allergy, and the results came back as negative. That does not mean the doctor tested you for gluten sensitivities. That can be done with an allergen test. But even without getting tested, you can tell if you are gluten sensitive simply by giving up all gluten for a week or two. If you have the sensitivity, you will feel much better, you will start losing weight, you will be able to sleep better, and your energy will noticeably increase.

FAT AND ENERGY

It always amazes me that when I ask my patients about what they eat, they give me all kinds of answers that cover a broad range of categories. Some patients have much better eating habits than others. But one thing most of them have in common is that they all include a large number of fat-free foods in their meals and snacks. It almost seems as if they're afraid of fat. My patients, along with much of the Western world, have been brainwashed to believe that fat is their enemy and must be avoided at all costs. They tend to look at me strangely when I tell them they must bring fat back into their diets. In fact, ideally you should consume a small amount of healthy fat with each meal and snack.

Healthy vs. Unhealthy Fats

What's important for you to understand first is that fat is not the enemy. For many years, the American public and—much more damaging—the American food producers bought into the premise that low-fat and no-fat foods were the ultimate answer to weight loss and a healthy heart. But as, Gary Taubes, author of a *New York Times* article called "What If It's All Been a Big Fat Lie?" stated, "the public health authorities told us unwittingly, but with the best of intentions, to eat precisely those foods that would make us fat, and we did. We ate more fat-free carbohydrates, which, in turn, made us hungrier and then heavier." Food manufacturers most often replaced fat with high-fructose corn syrup, which turned out to be much worse for us than the fat it replaced. As a society, we've been so worried about fat in the diet that nobody wants to put fat in anything or eat anything with fat in it.

Fortunately, the past few years have brought about a new understanding of the role of fats in our diet. What we have discovered is that certain classes of fat are very important to human health. They are critical for brain function, joint health, bone remodeling, great skin, and nutrient absorption. They help the body release CCK, which as we learned earlier, turns on the signals that tell you that you've eaten enough food. What we also now know is that it's not fat in general that's causing us problems, it's that most of us are ingesting too much of the wrong kinds of fat and too little of the right kinds. The best thing we can do is to learn to tell the difference.

One of the reasons the subject of fat is so confusing, is because there are so many different terms used when discussing fats. Here are some of the most common ways people refer to fats:

❖ **Essential fatty acid (EFA):** EFAs, which include omega-3s and omega-6s, are building blocks of the body, and they are necessary for human health. The body cannot make EFAs, so we must get them from the foods we eat (see page 45 for a list of EFA-containing foods). EFAs help not only slow down the rate at which glucose flows in the bloodstream, but also increase your body's metabolic rate and help burn fat.

❖ **Saturated fat:** The term *saturated fat* refers to a fat that has a large amount of hydrogen naturally attached to it—it is *saturated* with hydrogen. This molecular structure means that it is usually solid at room temperature. Saturated fat is found in animal fats and in some tropical oils such as coconut and palm.

❖ **Unsaturated fat:** This type of fat has fewer hydrogen atoms attached to it (which is why it is "*un*saturated"). It is derived from plant and some animal sources, especially fish, and is liquid at room temperature. There are two types of this fat: monounsaturated and polyunsaturated. Monounsaturated fats, including olive oil, peanut oil, flaxseed oil, and sesame oil, are typically liquid at room temperature, but can turn solid when refrigerated. Polyunsaturated fats remain liquid even when chilled.

❖ **Hydrogenated:** Another kind of fat that is saturated with hydrogen is called hydrogenated fat; however, this form of fat had hydrogen artificially added to it. This process is generally done to oils at extremely high temperatures to solidify them and give them longer shelf lives. Margarine is probably the most well-known hydrogenated product.

❖ **Trans fatty acid:** The process of hydrogenating fat causes it to change its molecular structure into what is called a trans fatty acid, which can be found in many commercially packaged goods, foods such as French fries from some fast food chains, other packaged snacks such as microwave popcorn, and in vegetable shortening and some margarine. If a label lists "partially hydrogenated vegetable oils," "hydrogenated vegetable oils," or "shortening," the product most likely contain trans fat. Both trans fats and hydrogenated fats can actually interfere with the body's ability to metabolize the good fats. Although there are many foods on the market now that are labeled "0 trans fats," they are still in a huge number of foods on the shelves and on restaurant menus. It may not be possible to entirely eliminate trans fats from your diet; the best strategy is to try to keep the proportion of EFAs and unsaturated fats higher than the trans fatty acids.

So how do you know which fats are good for you and which are not, which ones are energy drainers and which are energy producers? "Good" fats are those that are least saturated. When you see the words essential fatty acids, omega-3, omega-6, monounsaturated, and polyunsaturated, you can know that you're on the right track. The worst fats are the most saturated: hydrogenated, partially hydrogenated, and trans fats.

Omega-3 and Omega-6

I wanted to talk a little more about omega-3 and omega-6 fatty acids because they are so important to our health. Both of these are polyunsaturated fats, and both provide energy to our muscles and organs. They also play a role in brain function and help reduce inflammation in the body, thus leading to a lower risk of heart disease, cancer, arthritis, and other chronic conditions. Omega-6 has been shown to stimulate fat-burning tissue in the body, encouraging calories to be burned for energy instead of being stored as fat.

In February of 2009, the American Heart Association stated that omega-6 fatty acids are a beneficial part of a healthy eating plan, and they recommended that people aim for at least 5 to 10 percent of their calories from omega-6 fatty acids. They also said that most Americans already get enough omega-6 in foods they are currently eating, such as nuts, cooking oils, and salad dressings.

Your goal is to balance the amount of omega-3s and omega-6s you consume. Before the advent of so many processed foods, people consumed omega-3 and omega-6 fatty acids in roughly equal amounts. However, most Western civilizations now get far too much omega-6 and not enough of the omega-3. Because omega-6s are pro-inflammatory, this imbalance may explain the rise of such diseases as asthma, coronary heart disease, many forms of cancer, autoimmunity and neurodegenerative diseases, all of which are believed to stem from inflammation in the body. It also contributes to obesity and depression—two known energy zappers. The best way to cut down on omega-6 levels is by reducing consumption of processed and fast foods and polyunsaturated vegetable oils such as corn, sunflower, safflower, and cottonseed, and yes, even soy. (Learn more about soy on page 47.)

The best sources of omega-3s are fatty fish, but there are also many excellent plant-based sources. Omega-6s are found in leafy greens; however, the best source for them is the oil of certain plants. Following are lists of foods that will help you get your necessary helping of omega-3 and omega-6 fatty acids.

Best sources of omega-3:

Anchovies	Sardines
Atlantic Mackerel	Striped bass
Herring	Trout
Salmon	Tuna

Excellent food sources of omega-3s:

Avocados	Mustard seeds
Broccoli	Oregano
Brussels sprouts	Pumpkin seeds
Cabbage	Romaine lettuce
Cauliflower	Spinach
Cloves	Strawberries
Collard greens	Summer squash
Flaxseeds	Turnip greens
Green beans	Walnuts
Kale	Winter squash

Best sources of omega-6s:

Corn oil	Safflower oil
Cottonseed oil	Sunflower seeds
Grapeseed oil	Vegetable oil
Olive oil	Walnut oil
Pine nuts	Wheat germ oil
Pistachio nuts	

Try Eating with Your Hands

Many African chefs cook dishes, including messy barbecued chicken or beef, that are meant to be eaten with the hands, not with a knife and fork. They feel that eating with the hands gives you more satisfaction and more pleasure from your meals. They also use flavored oils instead of spices. They believe that the sense of smell goes to the hypothalamus (a center of the brain) and makes you feel satiated without having to eat so much (added to the fact that the oils contain the essential fatty acids we need for our health).

What We Do to Ourselves

When many of us shop, we look at what the farms are feeding the animals and the conditions under which those animals live. We don't want their soil to be contaminated with chemicals or heavy metals. We don't want the animals to be fed hormones or to have them live under stressful conditions. We know that can't be good for us. Yet many of us do to ourselves exactly what we don't want done to them.

When my daughter was turning ten, I decided to throw her a party. I invited several of her friends along with their parents. Before I knew it, the date of the party was upon me. I found myself completely unprepared. I needed to go shopping in the morning for the party that afternoon. I was running around in a frenzy, buying foods we almost never brought into the house—chips and dips, soda, candy, cookies, etc.—for several reasons. I didn't have much time to shop, and these foods were easy to find. I was trying to keep the cost of the party down, and these foods are relatively inexpensive. And I knew these were foods that everyone expects and enjoys at a birthday party. I guess I was just being a bit lazy, and I allowed myself to be careless in what I was serving. Even though I enjoyed myself at the party (and indulged in some of these less-than-healthy delights), I couldn't help thinking, *What if enemy aliens came to earth looking for food and saw how we were all filling our stomachs with sugar and fat and toxins? Would they still consider eating us for dinner?*

The foods that we are eating today are hitting us right in the gut, and many of us are suffering more than we should. In the next chapter, you'll find out just how our less-than-nutritious fare is giving us everything from agita to serious stomach problems, and what we can do about it.

THE ENERGY FURNACE
jump-start tips

1. **Got whole milk?** These days, because of the fear of fat in our country, many people drink only skim milk (if they drink milk at all). But with few exceptions, I suggest drinking whole milk instead. It has fewer carbohydrates in ratio to fat than skim. It's the ratio of the carbs to the proteins and the fats in the milk that make it a better choice. It does contain more fat, so you should consult with your health professional if you have, for instance, coronary artery disease, but in terms of both energy and weight loss, whole milk may actually be a better option. Milk is a kind of all-in-one package for a variety of nutrients our bodies need. It has protein, fat, carbohydrates, vitamins, and minerals. Sure, you can get all of these things from other places, but milk has them all conveniently packaged together for you. Some of the nutrient benefits contained in an 8-ounce glass of milk are: all three energy nutrients (proteins, carbs, and fats), calcium, potassium, and vitamins A, D, and B_{12}.

2. **Cut down on soy.** The soy industry has convinced the American public of this bean's benefits. However, soy can have a powerful influence on hormone production, especially estrogen. Studies have shown that babies who are fed only soy milk have 22,000

times as much estrogen in their systems as babies who have been breast-fed. That is the equivalent of giving them five birth-control pills a day. If adults took that many pills a day, they would suffer consequences including vomiting, abdominal pain, headaches, uterine bleeding, and blood clots. A little bit of soy is fine, and it can be hard to avoid because it is used as filler in many packaged products. But I would not suggest you have a soy latte every day, especially if you're also eating tofu and edamame (immature soybeans in the pod, which my children love, but I limit their consumption to a small serving once a week).

A large percentage of soy is genetically modified; it also has one of the highest percentages of pesticides in any food we eat. Over the years, many women have been convinced of the benefits of soy because of the low rates of breast cancer seen in many Asian countries, where soy consumption is much higher than in the United States. However, even those rates are rising rapidly. The 2009 Shanghai Breast Cancer Survival Study of more than 5,000 women diagnosed with breast cancer found that a high soy diet lowered the risk of recurrence and breast cancer death. However, the soy that women eat in China is in the form of lightly processed whole foods. The soy that most Americans eat is in the form of soy milk, soy supplements, and highly processed foods such as soy chips, cereals, and protein bars and most scientists suspect that the cancer protection is not the same from these products.

3. **Always eat breakfast.** Breakfast really *is* the most important meal of the day. This meal sets you up for the rest of the day's energy production. Studies show that people who eat breakfast every morning enjoy more energy and a better mood throughout the day. You should eat breakfast within one hour of waking up, and the meal should include protein and fat with no greater than 30 percent carbohydrates, which will help maintain steady glucose levels, lower insulin production, and result in less hunger and snacking throughout the rest of the day. If you're traveling

abroad and staying at any of the larger hotels, you will probably be offered an "American" breakfast. You will soon realize that it's a bit stingy: bread, jam, muffins, coffee. It's also mostly carbohydrates. This is *not* how most of the rest of the world eats breakfast. In the countryside and in the less touristy bed and breakfasts of most European countries, South America, Asia, and Africa, you'll find breakfasts that offer heartier fare, such as eggs, cheese, and yogurt, plus a variety of meats. This can be a healthier choice if you don't overindulge. If you're in a rush and don't have time for a full breakfast, have a protein shake. They come in a variety of flavors, and there are many quality brands available in health-food stores, specialty markets like Whole Foods and Trader Joe's, and many local supermarkets.

4. **Slow down.** If you eat too quickly, you don't give the brain time to send out satiety signals that say you're full. Take a "Zen" attitude toward your food—when you eat, sit down, take your time, honor your food, and let it nourish you. If at all possible, don't eat on the go. Sit at the dining room or kitchen table so that it feels like a real meal. Put your fork down between bites and thoroughly chew your food before you take the next one.

5. **Make your food beautiful.** Many cultures over the centuries have made beautiful bowls, glasses, and serving utensils. One of my patients told me that she puts liquids such as antioxidant drinks and green drinks in beautiful containers. It reminds her that life is beautiful and each day can be pleasurable. She also tries to place a flower near her plates or glasses. If she can't afford a fresh new flower, she uses a blade of grass, once again to remind her of how we live with nature. It is more appealing and therefore more pleasurable to eat in beautiful surroundings. This pleasure releases natural hormones, which produce satisfaction within the brain and allow you to feel fuller sooner.

6. **Use chopsticks and eat from small plates.** When my family and I were traveling in China, we ate at restaurants in several cities. Of course, we ate with chopsticks, which I highly recommend. No one in my family is an expert in their use, so we found that using chopsticks caused us to eat slowly and take small bites. That made the meal longer and the food more easily digestible. We also learned a lesson from the way the food was served. At our first dinner in China, the waiter brought over teacups and small plates. At first, we thought the plates were saucers for our tea cups, but they were not. The food there is served in a communal style: the dishes are placed on a lazy Susan and everyone takes their own portion. When our food was served, we did not start eating. We were waiting for our large dinner plates to arrive. It turned out there were no large dinner plates; you are supposed to serve yourself a little at a time on the small plates. At the beginning of our trip, we all loaded as much as possible onto our little plates. But by the end of our journey, we realized that by using the smaller plates we had become accustomed to eating much less food. Now when I make dinner at home, I serve on eight-inch salad plates instead of the standard ten-inchers, and my whole family has learned to eat less.

7. **Add a variety of gluten-free grains to your diet.** If you have gluten sensitivity or if you're curtailing your wheat consumption, you don't have to give up all grains. In fact, you should include grains in your diet as they are an excellent source of fiber. Here are some grains you can use as substitutions:

❖ Amaranth

❖ Barley

❖ Brown rice

❖ Buckwheat

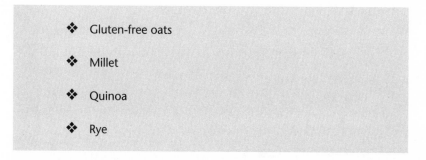

❖ Gluten-free oats

❖ Millet

❖ Quinoa

❖ Rye

You will be amazed at how much better you feel and how much more energy you have when you make the simple changes in your diet suggested in this chapter. However, you probably have a long history of eating improperly, which means that your digestive system may not be responding as well as it should. Now that you have a better idea of what and when to eat to increase your energy output, the next chapter will be of great help in keeping your digestive system in shape.

CHAPTER 3

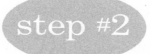

Get Your
Gut in Shape

Do you often feel inexplicably tired and run down?
Do you become easily irritated or depressed?
Is your thinking foggy or unclear?
Do you suffer from constipation?
Do you have skin eruptions and clogged pores?

Is your stomach making you tired? That may seem like an odd question, but if you answered "yes" to two or more of the questions above, you may be experiencing toxic overload, a condition that I consider to be one of the most frequent, yet least diagnosed, causes of fatigue. We are bombarded with environmental toxins on a daily basis (including pesticides, poor air quality, artificial chemicals, and foods with added hormones) that accumulate to create a toxic burden in our bodies. If that burden is allowed to remain in the body, it can become an ever-growing drain on many of our energy resources.

You may be surprised to find that your energy levels are tied into your gastrointestinal tract and that clearing toxins out of your body can help rejuvenate your entire system. Today, more than 75 percent of the population suffers from some type of gastrointestinal distress that can usually be traced back to food sensitivities or low enzyme activity inhibiting digestion. The foods you eat and your lifestyle in general can be causing your body a great deal of stress.

Unhealthy Diet, Unhealthy Gut

Did you know that during your lifetime, you will consume somewhere between 30 and 50 tons of food? Which do you think would be better for your GI health, 50 tons of nutrients, fiber, and antioxidants—or 50 tons of refined carbohydrates, additives, preservatives, hydrogenated fat, sugar, sugar, and more sugar? Unfortunately, the standard American diet (SAD) consists of far more of the latter. When we consume all those artificial substances—what we all know as junk food—it tends to just lie there in your stomach. We are not genetically programmed to easily digest this kind of food. It then places a significant burden on the digestive system. Bowel transit time is greatly reduced. Your gut becomes a breeding ground for "bad" bacteria, food allergies and sensitivities, and inflammation.

Problems of the Gut

Gastrointestinal (GI) complaints are one of the most common reasons that people seek out the advice of their physicians. What most of us don't realize, however, is that these "tummy aches" and feelings of discomfort can be the underlying sources of the fatigue that we are experiencing.

I have a colleague, also a doctor (although not an endocrinologist), who came to me to discuss her problems with fatigue. I asked the routine questions I ask every new patient, but when I started asking her about what she called "bathroom issues," she got embarrassed and tried to change the subject. "I'm here to find out why I'm so tired," she said. "There's no reason to discuss those kinds of bodily functions." And she's a doctor!

I'm always surprised by how little my patients know about the digestive process. I do understand that things having to do with the gut are usually considered somewhat gross, if not downright disgusting. Many people, particularly Americans, are embarrassed to talk about this part of their anatomy. They don't want to think about it, and they certainly don't want to discuss it.

It may surprise you that many other cultures are concerned and curious about their poo. In Africa, many people survive by being able to recognize what various species' poo looks like, which makes it possible to track them through the jungle or across the plains. When I was in Germany, I was surprised to see their "double-decker" toilets. They are actually called the reverse bowl design—the bowl is designed to hold the fecal matter out of the water prior to flushing. The lower level holds water, and that is where you pee. Many Germans and other Europeans look at their poo every time they go; they look at the texture, the color, and the quantity to diagnose how healthy they are.

Many times, problems with bowel movements are related to stress. While some people have more bowel movements when they are under stress, others find they become constipated. That is why some cultures strive to make the experience as comfortable and relaxing as possible. When I was in Japan, for instance, I went into a public bathroom. The lighting was dim, there was harpsichord music playing, everything was made of teak and bamboo, and there were bonsai trees all around. The atmosphere was soothing and calming.

Sometimes we think we're having digestive problems when we're really having time-management problems. I basically have to schedule time for myself in the morning. This seems to be more of a problem for women than for men—men just grab their newspapers and are behind closed doors for a half hour. Many women, however, have a hectic time in the morning getting the kids off to school and getting themselves off to work. You may have to wake up earlier or wait until everyone else has left the house, but just be sure to give yourself enough time for your body to function the way it should.

How the Gut Works

It's really important that you understand the gut and how it works, because if you can fix what is wrong with your gut, many other things—including fatigue—may be fixed as well.

First, here is some basic anatomy: An adult's digestive tract, which is about 30 feet (9 meters) long, is a tubelike system in which food enters through the mouth, passes through a long cylinder, and exits the body as feces through the anus. There are muscles in the walls of our digestive organs (including the esophagus, stomach, and intestines) that keep food moving along through the system, where it is broken down into nutrients that can be absorbed by the body. There are other organs, such as the liver and the pancreas, that are also a part of the digestive process.

Digestion, the process by which food is broken down into simple chemical compounds that can be absorbed and used as nutrients or eliminated by the body, is one of the most energy-consuming functions of the human body. Food must be broken down all the way to its individual molecules to be useable. Our cells cannot absorb any of food's nutritional benefits until it has been "digested," meaning, converted into energy and other useful components, which can then be absorbed into the bloodstream and distributed throughout the body. We must have sufficient amounts of energy available if we are to eliminate the toxins from the body. When there is any kind of disturbance within the digestive process, there is also a resultant disturbance in energy production.

When patients come into my office complaining of fatigue, I often surprise them by asking if they have had any stomach issues as well. "Yes, I have!" they say. "How did you know?" I know because stomach problems, especially the three common issues described below, can be the cause of the fatigue the patient is experiencing.

Dysbiosis

The human intestinal tract is inhabited by thousands of strains of bacteria, some beneficial, some harmful. The balance between these strains can have a huge impact on whether a person feels well or ill. When the intestines are healthy and in balance and everything is functioning smoothly, they are described as being in a state of *symbiosis*. When there is an imbalance of the bacteria in the digestive tract, an overgrowth of yeast, or the presence of viruses or parasites in the intestines, they are described as being in a state of *dysbiosis*. The way I often describe it is that we have houseguests all the time. Some are welcome, some are not welcome. When there are too many unwelcome guests, we have dysbiosis.

Some symptoms or warning signs of dysbiosis include:

❖ Chronic unexplained fatigue

❖ Leaky gut syndrome

❖ Irritable bowel syndrome

❖ Acne, eczema, and other skin problems

❖ Bad breath and gum disease

❖ Chronic yeast problems and candida overgrowth

❖ Acid reflux

❖ Frequent colds, flus, and infections

An imbalance in the body's intestinal flora can come from many sources. Many of these microbes simply die off with age. Stress, illness, and certain medications all take their toll on the "good guys" that live within us. So does a poor diet, and we'll talk more about food and GI health starting on page 58.

The first step in treating dysbiosis is to see your doctor or health professional to determine which organisms are causing the dysbiotic condition, and what the best treatment may be. Some people may be required to change their diet and lifestyle habits.

Dysbiosis on the Yangtze

My family and I were traveling on a month-long journey through several eastern Asian countries. Unfortunately, my husband got a bad case of food poisoning in Kazakhstan near the border of Uzbekistan. I tried to handle it with antibiotics and Western medicine techniques, but after many days, he still wasn't any better. We continued traveling, though, and were on a boat on the Yangtze River when I suggested he go see the Chinese doctor on board for some acupuncture. My husband was skeptical, but he was so weak at this point (he had lost almost 30 pounds in a little more than a week) he was willing to try anything. When the acupuncturist inserted two needles above his knees, my husband tried frantically to communicate that the doctor, who didn't speak any English, must be mistaken, that he wasn't having trouble with his knees. Somehow, the doctor was able to persuade my husband to stay. The doctor then inserted two needles in his lower abdominal area and within minutes, the gastroenteritis (irritation of the intestinal tract) disappeared. My husband's infection had actually been cured by the antibiotics I had given him, but once that kind of diarrhea starts, the electrical system in your body goes haywire, and you get a disruption of the homeostasis (equilibrium) of the gut. The acupuncture repaired the electrical current, which is why it worked. My husband, who had been miserable for over a week, was not only cured, he felt energized and rejuvenated. I've always been an advocate of acupuncture, but now I am a devotee (and so is my husband).

Candida

It always amazes me when a patient with recurrent vaginal infections is surprised to find out she also has yeast growing in her gut. If you look at the causes for these vaginal infections, it should make sense to you—causes such as too much caffeine, not enough sleep, excessive alcohol consumption, smoking tobacco (or something else), heavy metal contamination, and too much acidity in the diet, not enough alkalinity. In other words, an unbalanced life. Why would this tiny yeast organism want to live *only* in the vagina when it has the entire intestinal tract to hang out in?

One specific form of dysbiosis is candidiasis, the overgrowth of a yeastlike fungus that may thrive in the intestinal tract, mouth, skin, and vagina. There are a wide variety of symptoms that may include fatigue, "brain fog," and skin conditions such as eczema and psoriasis. *Candida albicans* and other species of yeast are normally found in the body but become a problem when there is an overgrowth. The normal balance of organisms in the intestinal tract is thrown off and there are too many of one kind of organism and not enough of another living on top of each other in the same area. It's like poor urban planning: too many buildings and not enough parks.

In some cases, the candida overgrowth in the intestines can penetrate the intestinal wall, causing the yeast and other unwanted particles to be absorbed into the body. This is thought to activate the immune system, resulting in fatigue, headache, mood swings, poor memory and concentration, and cravings for sweets.

Candida causes a craving for sweets because it thrives on carbohydrates. It is kept alive by sugar, so naturally it sends out the message "Feed me!" and demands even more sugar. High consumption of sugar, white flour, and all sorts of junk food perpetuate the overgrowth of candida and keep it going. If you've ever had a yeast infection on your skin—jock itch, for instance, is a yeast infection—you know how uncomfortable it is. It becomes inflamed, and you want to scratch it all the time. This same thing is happening inside your body when you have a yeast infection.

Candida can also be caused by long-term antibiotic use, too much alcohol, and chronic stress, which suppresses the immune system. In fact, any time you are ill, your immune system is temporarily compromised, and candida can easily take the opportunity to proliferate.

It is sometimes difficult to diagnose a candida infection. While vaginal yeast infections are fairly easy to spot, overgrowth within the GI tract is often unrecognized. It doesn't always present itself as bloat or diarrhea. When a patient comes in with symptoms such as fatigue and brain fog, the doctor doesn't immediately think of candida. But there are tests that your doctor can perform (see Chapter 9) to measure the amount of candida in your system and detect elevated levels in your intestinal tract.

Once you have a candida overgrowth, you are likely to get it again. The best defense against candida overgrowth is modify your diet to reduce its sugar content. That means limiting soft drinks, juices, breads, pastries, candies, cakes, cupcakes, and so on. Be careful to read all labels as there are often hidden sugars in products such as salad dressing, ketchup, and barbecue sauce.

Your diet should include lean proteins and high fiber, as well as spices that have antifungal properties such as oregano, thyme, garlic, onion, rosemary, and sage.

From Dr. Eva's Files

Wendy came in to see me because she was experiencing breast tenderness and thought she might be in perimenopause. She was also frequently fatigued. I examined her and could see that she was bloated. I asked her about her bowel habits, and she told me she was often constipated. All these symptoms began to make me think she might have a candidia overgrowth. When we tested her, it turned out that she not only had candidiasis, she had mercury toxicity as well. As a matter of fact, research shows that there is a link between metal toxicity and candida yeast infections, and that 80 percent of individuals who had candida yeast infections also tested high on mercury levels in their systems. When there is toxic metal overload in the intestine, the intestinal lining produces extra mucus to block metals from being absorbed into the bloodstream. The problem is that this mucus creates an environment that lacks oxygen, thus encouraging bacteria and fungilike organisms such as candida yeast to grow out of control.

Wendy, who was originally from Singapore, had been told several years earlier that she had a candida overgrowth, but never did a detox. She ate a lot of fish, but never connected her fish consumption to her candidiasis. I gave her oral chelation therapy using an amino acid compound to tightly bind to heavy metals and transport them out of the body, generally through the urine, and placed her on an anticandida diet and supplements for six weeks. All of her symptoms improved, and her breast tenderness disappeared.

Leaky Gut Syndrome

Leaky gut syndrome (LGS) occurs when the lining of the intestines is weakened to the point that their contents can leak out and enter the bloodstream, causing a variety of health problems from fatigue to food sensitivities to skin rashes to migraines. Although the cause of LGS is not really known, it has at times been attributed to allergies, exposure to toxins (which would in turn cause the toxins to leak into the bloodstream), and poor dietary choices.

The symptoms of leaky gut syndrome can include abdominal pain, heartburn, fatigue, insomnia, bloating, anxiety, gluten intolerance, malnutrition, muscle cramps and pains, poor exercise tolerance, and food allergies. There are many lifestyle and dietary recommendations that can help improve LGS, including:

❖ Eliminate alcohol consumption during the GI healing phase.

❖ Completely avoid use of aspirin and NSAIDs.

❖ Avoid constipation—eat plenty of fiber-rich foods and drink eight glasses of water per day.

❖ Control stress (you can use biofeedback, deep breathing, yoga, meditation, proper sleep, etc.).

❖ Avoid excess consumption of coffee, tea, and soda.

❖ Consume organic fruits and vegetables and free-range meat and poultry whenever possible.

❖ Eat five to nine servings of fresh fruits and vegetables daily.

❖ Avoid sugar and artificially sweetened products. Replace sugar with stevia or xylitol (see page 69).

❖ Concentrate on fish and foods high in omega-3 fatty acids such as salmon, mackerel, and sardines.

It is not always easy to see the connections of various maladies going in your body. Forty-five-year-old Bonnie was so fatigued that she could barely drag herself into my office. For the last two decades, she had suffered from sinusitis (inflammation of the inner lining of the sinus) at least four times a year. She constantly felt pressure like, as she said, "a truck sitting on my face." That meant she was taking antibiotics at least four times a year. It would clear up her sinuses, but it would also completely destroy the homeostasis of her gut. The antibiotics would kill off the good guys and the bad guys equally. Without those good bacterial warriors, the bad guys could simply move in and take over. Because of this, she was destroying the lining of her intestines, and she developed leaky gut syndrome. We wanted to find out what was causing her sinuses to become inflamed in the first place, so we performed a food allergy panel on her to find any sensitivities she might have. These kinds of sensitivities don't just cause inflammation in the gut, they cause inflammation along every mucosal area you have—including the nose and throat.

We found that Bonnie had several food sensitivities, especially to aspergillus, a fungus that's mostly found in wine, which contributed to her bloat and fatigue. She eliminated the wine and the other foods to which she was sensitive, and followed the recommendations for lifestyle and dietary changes on page 81 to restore her gut health. She is no longer fatigued, and she only occasionally suffers from sinusitis anymore.

Irritable Bowel Syndrome

The best description of bloating, one of the most common symptoms of irritable bowel syndrome (IBS), came from a patient of mine who said, "When I walk into a room, I feel as if my stomach walks in first." When people are bloated, the mere pressure against their diaphragm inhibits them from breathing deeply and causes them to have pressure against their lungs. They feel as if they're carrying around a dead weight, which is exhausting. IBS is not life-threatening, but it can cause great fatigue and negatively impact the quality of everyday life.

It is estimated that IBS affects 10 to 20 percent of the American population, with women 20 to 40 years old accounting for the majority of patients. It is one of the most common gastrointestinal disorders seen in doctors' offices. About 12 percent of all primary-care doctor visits are IBS related, making IBS one of the top ten reasons people go to the doctor. It is also one of the leading causes of missed workdays in the United States, second only to the common cold.

IBS is considered a syndrome and not a disease, therefore there is no specific test for it, and it is generally diagnosed after other disorders have been ruled out. Symptoms include fatigue, chronic abdominal pain or cramping, and major disturbance of bowel functioning. People with IBS may suffer with bouts of urgent diarrhea, episodes of chronic constipation, or a pattern of alternating between the two. Sometime you have neither and all you have is bloating.

One of the major triggers for the onset and exacerbation of IBS is stress. In fact, it is commonly believed that IBS is a disorder of the interaction between the brain and the gastrointestinal tract. Just think about a time when you were facing a stressful situation—having to speak before a large number of people, for instance, or just before a big game—and you suddenly had the urgent need for a bathroom break. People with IBS frequently also suffer from anxiety or depression as well. Infections of the gastrointestinal tract, as well as yeast overgrowth and/or depletion of beneficial gut flora can also lead to IBS.

What's necessary to understand about the diagnosis of IBS is that it is actually a diagnosis of exclusion. What that means is that when everything else has been ruled out as a source of chronic abdominal pain or bloating or alteration in bowel habits and doctors can't find the source, then it's diagnosed as IBS.

IBS and Gallstones

One particularly disturbing study showed that the rate of unnecessary gallbladder removal is significantly higher among IBS patients than non-IBS patients. Many IBS patients do suffer from gallstones (small, hard "pebbles" that form inside the gallbladder). These patients—and their doctors—often assume that abdominal pain they're experiencing comes from these stones. They then have the gallbladder removed, only to find that the abdominal pain returns, which means that it was not being caused by gallstones after all.

I had a patient who had been suffering from chronic stomach pain for months. She was young and slender and yet was always complaining about being tired. She had a fast-paced job and was well connected in society. In an effort to solve her discomfort, she had an ultrasound done. The radiologist said she had gallstones and sent her for a surgical consultation. The surgeon looked at the ultrasound results and advised the surgery to remove the source of her misery, the gallbladder. After the operation, the surgeon called me, perplexed, and explained that this patient in fact had gallbladder agenisis—meaning that there was no gallbladder to be found. Apparently, she was born without one, which does occur in a small minority of people. Both the radiologist and the surgeon had misdiagnosed the situation. What they had seen on her X-rays turned out to be calcified feces that looked like gallstones. The chance of being born without a gallbladder is so rare, it did not enter either one of their minds, which puts into perspective just how IBS can disguise itself as any number of things.

The recommendations for treating IBS are similar to those for leaky gut syndrome. However, because it's not clear what causes irritable bowel syndrome, treatment focuses on the relief of symptoms so that you can live as normally as possible. In many cases, you can learn to manage stress and make changes in your diet and lifestyle to successfully control mild signs and symptoms of irritable bowel syndrome. If your problems are more severe, you may need more than lifestyle changes. You may want to try:

❖ **Eliminating high-gas foods:** If you have bothersome bloating or are passing considerable amounts of gas, your doctor may suggest that you cut out such items as carbonated beverages, salads, raw fruits and vegetables, especially cabbage, broccoli and cauliflower.

❖ **Anticholinergic medications:** Some people need medications that affect certain activities of the autonomic nervous system (anticholinergics) to relieve painful bowel spasms. These may be helpful for people who have bouts of diarrhea but can worsen constipation.

❖ **Medications for constipation:** There are two drugs, Zelnorm and Amitiza, used to treat IBS with constipation as their main bowel problem. These two drugs are used to calm the stomach down in the same way that Prozac is used to treat depression and other conditions within the brain.

❖ **Antidepressant medications:** If your symptoms include pain or depression, your doctor may recommend a tricyclic antidepressant or a selective serotonin reuptake inhibitor (SSRI). These medications help relieve depression as well as inhibit the activity of neurons that control the intestines.

One final reason that IBS causes fatigue has to do with something called glutamic acid, an excitatory neurotransmitter that increases the firing of neurons in the central nervous system. It is converted into either glutamine or gamma-aminobutyric acid (GABA), two other amino acids that help pass messages to the brain. GABA is a natural calming agent in the brain that is manufactured from amino acids and glucose. It is sometimes called "nature's Valium" because when there are too many excitatory neurotransmitters firing in the brain, GABA will be sent out to try to calm things down. Many sedative and tranquilizing drugs act by enhancing the effects of GABA. When the gut becomes irritated and inflamed, there is less glutamic acid available, which means there is less GABA produced, which leads to food cravings, and insomnia, as well as feeling stressed, emotional, restless, hungry, and fatigued. This can be tested by stool as well as blood and urine analysis.

TOXINS, TOXINS EVERYWHERE

Think about some of the machines you have. If you want your air conditioner to keep you cool, you clean or change its filter every so often. You change the oil in your car so that the engine runs more efficiently. You keep your computer running smoothly by preventing it from getting dusty. You're constantly removing the dirt, dust, and gunk that keeps these machines from working at their highest efficiency.

Toxins are your body's dirt, dust, and gunk, and they can do damage in several ways. They are poisonous to the cells themselves, they disrupt the metabolism of cells, they interfere with the digestive process, and, like dirt that gets into machinery, they cause your body to have to exert more energy just to function properly. In other words, toxins make you tired.

There are three types of toxins that can be causing you fatigue:

❖ **Internal toxins:** These come from the overgrowth of organisms that are harbored within us, such as bacteria, yeast, and fungi. Bacteria flourish on what you feed them. If you feed them fresh, whole foods, good bacteria will grow. If you feed them junk food, bad bacteria will thrive and begin to produce nasty toxins. Toxins can come from metabolic reactions within the body (which produce carbon dioxide, ammonia, and hormones); from undigested food; and from both physical and emotional stress, including trauma, abuse, and taxing relationships with a spouse, relative, co-worker, friend, etc.

❖ **Environmental toxins:** At this point, if you live in the world and you're eating and breathing, you are likely to be exposed to varying degrees of environmental toxins. However, you will have a higher exposure to these types of toxins if you live in a large city, or close to a factory; if you're exposed to auto exhaust; if you work in a Laundromat or dry cleaning facility or are consistently around cleaning products; if you work as a painter and are exposed to solvents; if you're a gardener or landscaper and you're around pesticides all the time; or if you've had long-term exposure to heavy metals such as lead, mercury, arsenic, or cadmium.

❖ **Lifestyle toxins:** These are toxins we're exposed to because of the lifestyles we choose. These include nicotine, caffeine, and alcohol; over-the-counter, prescription, and recreational drugs; foods that contain additives, preservatives, hormones, and antibiotics; and foods that have been processed and refined.

The problem is not only that we have been exposed to all of these toxins, but also that toxins can remain in the body for many years. Many of the toxins that invade our bodies are fat soluble, which means that they aren't flushed out of our system via urine; instead they remain behind in our tissues and our bodies don't have the necessary mechanisms to remove them in a timely manner.

I try to explain to my patients who say, "I only smoke when I drink" or "I don't drink *that* much alcohol" or "I only drink caffeinated beverages before 3:00 P.M." that I would much rather they eliminate these lifestyle choices altogether. If they can't do that, it is good to limit their exposure. Also it's important for all of us to remember that as we age, we accumulate more and more toxins and the body has to work harder and harder to get rid of them.

More Reasons to Eat Protein at Every Meal

Here's another reason to eat more protein: it is rich in an enzyme called glutathione, a powerful antioxidant and a key nutrient for the detox process. Glutathione is made in the body from the amino acids glycine, cysteine, and glutamic acid, which you get from protein foods.

Glutathione is also found in some fruits and vegetables, including grapefruit, oranges, strawberries, tomatoes, cantaloupe, watermelon, broccoli, spinach, asparagus, and zucchini. Artichokes and watercress are especially good for you, as both of these foods have been shown to support liver function and promote the detox process.

THE DETOX SOLUTION

When Robyn came to my office, I was immediately struck by her beauty—although she looked a bit drawn and sallow. As we sat and talked, Robyn revealed that was 27 and a model whose career took her all over the world. She had been exhausted for several years, but she believed that the cause of her troubles was jet lag and long hours of shooting for the camera. She decided to slow down and stay in one city for a while to recover from her fatigue. Despite this lifestyle change, she seemed no better after several months, and her bookings started to drop off. She became concerned and so finally saw her doctor. Her physical exam and her routine lab results, were both normal.

Still, she wasn't feeling well, so she came to see me. She was surprised when I asked her certain questions, and I was surprised at some of the answers she gave me. She thought it was normal to have a bowel movement once a week. She thought it was normal to feel bloated all the time. She thought the rash on the back of her arms was a normal consequence of dry skin due to all the airplanes she had been on. And she thought it was normal to drink approximately 15 diet sodas a day to keep thin. Over time, she said, her weight had slowly crept up despite the fact that she kept cutting calories. So she continued to compensate by adding more sodas to her daily diet.

When I got the results of Robyn's stool analysis, it appeared that her intestinal balance was upside down. She had an overgrowth of organisms that shouldn't have been there and not enough of the ones that should have been. She hadn't realized all the mayhem that the artificial sweetener in all those sodas had caused. I told her I had a simple cure for her—give up diet soda. After one month with no diet sodas and a strict detoxification regimen her rash subsided, her bowel movements increased (although it took several months for her to have them daily), her weight normalized, her bloat disappeared, and her energy started to improve. She went back to work, flying all over the planet, *not* drinking diet sodas, and getting moe agency bookings than ever before.

Sweet and Sugar-Free

Most people in the Western world love their sugar. Eastern countries don't use anywhere near the amount of sugar we do. People in Asian countries don't appear to have a sweet tooth except for the occasional piece of fruit. Here in the United States, however, we love sweet foods and beverages even though we know sugar is bad for us, so we're constantly looking for that magical sugar substitute. One of the most ubiquitous is an additive called aspartame, which is found in more than 6,000 foods and beverages. However, many recent studies have found that aspartame causes side effects including headaches, insomnia, mood alterations, and gastrointestinal problems. In fact, a study published in 2008 in the *European Journal of Clinical Nutrition* found that aspartame may inhibit the ability of enzymes in the brain to function normally, and may lead to neurodegeneration (loss of function of the neurons).

What is a sweet-lover to do? There are two alternatives that are safe to use. One is Stevia, an herb in the chrysanthemum family which grows wild as a small shrub in parts of Paraguay and Brazil. It's not only a no-calorie sweetener, it's an antioxidant as well. My personal favorite, however, is xylitol. It prevents tooth decay, rather than causing it, which is why it is often used in sugar-free gum as well as oral hygiene products such as toothpaste, fluoride tablets and mouthwashes. Studies have shown that xylitol may also help control oral infections of candida yeast. Derived from the bark of the birch tree, it is lower in calories than sugar, with 9.6 calories per teaspoon, as compared to one teaspoon of sugar, which has 15 calories.

The purpose of detoxification is to cleanse the body of internal impurities, which if left to thrive could cause deterioration and disease. Taking steps to thoroughly detox the body will restore your physical and emotional energy, increase your mental stamina, improve your digestive processes, aid with weight loss, and help you feel and look much healthier.

Detoxification is the metabolic process by which toxins are changed into less toxic or more easily excretable substances. It's the method by which the body gets rid of the gunk and the sludge and the waste materials that, if left alone, would slow us down, tire us out, and do us harm.

The body does have several built-in filtration systems, including the intestines, the kidneys, and the skin. But the most important system we have is the liver, which filters out and transforms toxins that have entered the bloodstream into harmless substances that can be eliminated through the urine. But when there is an overabundance of toxins, the liver and the body's other filtration systems have difficulty doing their jobs. Not only do you end up with indigestion, stomach bloat, and myriad other health problems, the excess toxins can cause hormonal changes as well. You can end up with worsening PMS and even premature menopause. That's because the liver produces proteins called binding globulins that are released into the bloodstream. Picture them as tiny taxis transporting hormones to their ultimate destinations. When the liver gets filled with toxins, they rudely cut in line and bind onto these globulin taxis, aggressively preventing the hormones from getting where they need to go. The liver gets sidetracked trying to eliminate the poisonous troublemakers, which disrupts your hormones, which then creates fatigue, low energy, mood changes, and a weakened immune system.

The best way to start getting your gut in shape is to detoxify, which is the process of eliminating the build-up of wastes and toxins from the body. Many people believe that fasting is the best way to detox the body. However, studies have shown that fasting depletes the body of essential nutrients and can have many adverse health effects, including decreased energy production. Other studies have shown that efficient functioning of the liver's detoxification system requires adequate protein. Also, it appears that high carbohydrate intake reduces the ability of certain detoxification enzymes to work effectively. So the way to bolster your natural detoxification system is not to stop eating, but to follow the Fatigue Solution program, consuming more protein and focusing on healthy carbohydrates.

TOXICITY AND INFLAMMATION QUESTIONNAIRE: GENERAL SIGNS AND SYMPTOMS

Inflammation is the immune system's response to foreign invaders, or what it perceives to be foreign invaders. The more toxins and artificial food substances you introduce into your digestive system, the more inflammation will also be introduced.

Since there are so many different types of stomach ailments and diseases, you should always visit your health professional if you are having problems in order to rule out any serious disorders. This questionnaire identifies signs and symptoms that can help your doctor address the underlying cause of your GI-related illness. It is to be completed before you go to see your doctor so that you can best describe your symptoms during your visit (this questionnaire is used with permission from *Pillars of G.I. Health: Physician Road Map,* Ortho Molecular Products).

Point Scale:

0 = never or almost never have the symptom

1 = occasionally have it, effect is not severe

2 = occasionally have it, effect is severe

3 = frequently have it, effect is not severe

4 = frequently have it, effect is severe

HEAD

___ Headaches

___ Dizziness

___ Insomnia

___ Faintness

____ TOTAL

EARS

___ Itchy ears

___ Ringing in ears/loss of hearing

___ Earaches/ear infections

___ Drainage from ear

____ TOTAL

EYES
___ Bags or dark circles under eyes
___ Watery of itchy eyes
___ Swollen, reddened, or sticky eyelids
___ Blurred or tunnel vision (excluding near- or far-sightedness)
____ TOTAL

NOSE
___ Stuffy nose
___ Sinus congestion, sinus infection
___ Constant sneezing
___ Hay fever/allergies
___ Excess mucus formation
____ TOTAL

MOUTH/THROAT
___ Chronic coughing
___ Sore throat, hoarseness, loss of voice
___ Gagging, frequent need to clear throat
___ Swollen tongue, gums, or lips
___ Canker sores, mouth ulcers
____ TOTAL

HEART
___ Chest pain
___ Irregular or skipped heartbeat
___ Rapid of pounding heartbeat
____ TOTAL

LUNGS
___ Asthma, bronchitis
___ Chest congestion
___ Shortness of breath
___ Difficulty breathing
____ TOTAL

SKIN
___ Acne or brown "age/liver spots"
___ Hives, rashes, cysts, boils
___ Eczema or psoriasis
___ Hair loss, thinning
___ Body odor
___ Excessive sweating
____ TOTAL

JOINTS/MUSCLES
___ Pain or aches in joints or lower back
___ Stiffness or limitation of movement
___ Arthritis
___ Pain or aches in muscles
____ TOTAL

MENTAL/EMOTIONAL
___ Poor memory
___ Difficulty concentrating
___ Mood swings
___ Depression
___ Anxiety, fear, or nervousness
___ Anger, irritability, or aggressiveness
___ Insomnia
____ TOTAL

ENERGY LEVEL
___ Fatigue/low energy
___ Restlessness
___ Hyperactivity
___ Feeling of weakness
____ TOTAL

WEIGHT
___ Underweight
___ Overweight
___ Difficulty losing weight
___ Crave certain foods
____ TOTAL

DIGESTIVE TRACT
___ Nausea, vomiting
___ Diarrhea
___ Constipation
___ Bloated feeling
___ Belching, passing gas
___ Heartburn
___ Intestinal/stomach pain
____ TOTAL

OTHER
___ PMS
___ Frequent colds, flu
___ Chemical or environmental sensitivities
___ Food allergies/sensitivities
____ TOTAL

Please add the numbers from each section and write the section total in the spaces provided, then add all the section totals together and put that total in the space below.

____ GRAND TOTAL

Interpreting your GRAND TOTAL Toxicity Score:

15 or lower: You have a low level of inflammation.
16 to 49: You have a moderate level of inflammation.
50 or higher: You have a high level of inflammation.

PROBIOTICS: THE FRIENDLY BACTERIA

One way to help manage problems of the gut is by supporting the intestinal flora through the use of probiotics. Probiotic literally means "for life." The World Health Organization (WHO) defines probiotics as "live microorganisms, which when given in adequate amounts, confer a health benefit on the host." In other words, probiotics are living bacteria that are similar to the friendly bacteria found in the human intestinal system. They live symbiotically in the gut, meaning they form a give-and-take relationship where they help us fight off the bad guys in return for a warm place to live. There are a few common probiotics, such as *Saccharomyces boulardii,* are yeasts, which are different from bacteria.

Probiotics work by constantly adjusting the intestinal immune environment to help correct the balance between beneficial and harmful bacteria and to prevent disease-causing bacteria from attacking and colonizing the gut. They restrict the overgrowth of harmful bacteria and promote the growth of helpful bacteria, which in turn enhances digestion and absorption of nutrients.

Most often, the bacteria come from two groups: *Lactobacillus* or *Bifidobacterium*. Within each group, there are different species, for example, *Lactobacillus acidophilus* (simply known as acidophilus) and *Bifidobacterium bifidus*; and within each species, there are different strains or varieties. Some of these probiotics are colonizing bacteria, which means that they are very "sticky" and adhere to the wall of the bowel. Others, such as the species *bulgarica,* are transient; it moves through the bowel and sweeps away some of the pathogens that may be harmful to us. In its wake it leaves a healthier, pinker colon. You can tell if you have enough of these bacteria by doing a stool test, which can show the different strains and quantities of them. In that way, you can replace exactly what you need.

One thing to note about stool tests: there are tests and there are *tests*. Patients often tell me that they've already had "a complete workup" from their regular physician. However, what they don't realize is that most doctors only do standard testing, which means they are looking for disease states and disease bacteria such as salmonella, shigella, and *Helicobacter pylori* (H pylori), which causes gastritis. They do not look for the full spectrum of organisms—bacteria, yeast, and parasites—that can live in our bodies. That's why patients can go to doctor after doctor without finding out what's really wrong with them. What I recommend is a comprehensive stool test that does test for the full spectrum. That's how we can detect organisms that are not deadly but that affect your quality of life. So when a patient tells me she's been tested, she usually means she's had the standard test done.

A variety of strains of bacteria inhabit different sections of the GI tract. Certain strains digest sugars, fats, or proteins. Other strains break down carbohydrates. Some species manufacture B vitamins and vitamin K. The good bacteria help prevent bloating, gas, and yeast overgrowth by controlling the pH level, or acidity, of the intestines. Probiotics helps facilitate proper hormone balance as well, which can help relieve symptoms of PMS, perimenopause, and menopause. It's virtually impossible to do harm by taking too much of this supplement. In fact, I recommend probiotics as part of a daily and indefinite routine. I'd rather you take a probiotic every day than a multivitamin.

As you can see from the list of symptoms above for dysbiosis, fatigue is right up there. The use of probiotics is one way to keep the digestive process healthy and effective, which is an important aspect of fighting fatigue. Any damage to the digestive tract will noticeably zap your energy, because it means that you are not able to properly absorb the important nutrients from the food you eat, which is, of course, the fuel your energy furnace. Even patients with chronic fatigue syndrome have reported that probiotics improved fatigue levels, according to a 2009 study published in the *Nutrition Journal*.

Antibiotics and Probiotics

Antibiotics are used to kill off "bad" bacteria that may be causing the body harm. Unfortunately, they often kill off good bacteria in the gut at the same time. Antibiotics frequently cause diarrhea as well when they disturb the natural balance of bacteria in your gut, causing certain bacteria to multiply far beyond normal numbers. Antibiotic diarrhea affects up to one in five people receiving antibiotic therapy. Researchers are now beginning to advocate the use of probiotics to restore the gut flora during and after a course of antibiotics. In fact, in 2008 researchers at the Albert Einstein College of Medicine recommended that doctors prescribe probiotics at the same time they prescribe antibiotics. They also noted that the effects of probiotics are short-lived, so they should be taken throughout the course of antibiotics. They recommended doses of at least 10 billion colony-forming units (CFUs) per day for adults.

How to Choose a Probiotic

Choosing a probiotic supplement can be tricky because there are many different strains and many different dosages on the market. When you're looking for a good probiotics, be sure to check the label. It should identify the strain of bacteria contained in the product and how many bacteria, or CFUs, there are in each recommended dose. The two most common strains you will find are *Lactobacillus* and *Bifodabacterium,* which includes the best-known *L. acidophilus* strain. A good place to find studies on various probiotic strains is the Web site www.PubMed.gov.

Probiotics come in many forms, including chewable tablets, capsules, powders, liquids, and foods such as yogurt and dairy drinks. Most experts agree that the form you take doesn't matter as long as there are enough live organisms to begin growing in the intestine. Unfortunately, experts do not agree on the effective dose, and numbers vary widely from 50 million to as many as 1 trillion live cells per dose. Unless you're getting diarrhea or abdominal pain, I believe that taking more probiotic is more beneficial than taking less. According to the World Health Organization, probiotics packaging should contain the following information:

❖ Strain—What probiotic is inside

❖ CFU—How many live microorganisms are in each serving

❖ Expiration date—Probiotics are not very effective past the expiration date

❖ Suggested serving size—How much you take

❖ Proper storage conditions—Does it need to be refrigerated? Kept at room temperature?

❖ Corporate contact information—Where can you go for more information

There is no standard labeling requirement to make it easier to choose a probiotic product. The word *probiotic* on the label is not enough information to tell whether a given product will be effective for a particular health concern. As of now there is no consistent way to tell if you're buying the most effective product for the problem you're looking to solve. The best answer at this time is probably to consult with your health professional to find which product(s) he or she recommends. Or you can check out a book called the *NutriSearch Comparative Guide to Nutritional Supplements* (professional version) by Lyle MacWilliam, which ranks supplements from zero to five for effectiveness and how beneficial they are.

Probiotics and Yogurt

One issue that confuses many consumers is that of probiotics in yogurt. As opposed to what most television and print advertising would have you believe, all yogurt contains live active cultures. The people who manufacture "probiotic" yogurt, however, claim that the bacteria in their products are more likely to survive digestion and make it to the colon. Many of these companies have trademarked the bacteria they use, and they believe their studies justify their claims of superiority to regular yogurt.

Experts are divided on the issue of whether probiotic yogurt is more effective than regular yogurt, and more studies need to be done comparing the two. While it's true that any yogurt with live cultures might ease some digestive ills, that doesn't necessarily mean that products labeled probiotic yogurt are superior. One thing to be aware of is other ingredients that may be added to these products, such as high levels of sweeteners like high-fructose corn syrup and/or sugar. More commercial yogurts and yogurt drinks usually have the most sugar, so you may want to stick with unsweetened natural yogurt. Try adding fresh fruit or a touch of honey for sweetness.

This is where making a judgment call comes in. If you're already taking several supplements a day, you may not want to add another one. Adding a container of yogurt into your diet may be the solution for you. Yogurt makes a great breakfast, especially if you don't have a lot of time in the morning. Get a plain yogurt and add a small amount of fruit, or try some Greek yogurt. You can't really overdose on probiotics, so if you want to eat yogurt in addition to taking a probiotic supplement, that's fine, too.

If you want to get rid of the "F" word, one of the best things you can do for yourself is to preserve your gut health. When I explain this to my patients, they often want me to tell them the very best things they can eat to keep them healthy. What I tell them is this: Take the old-fashioned approach. Ask your grandmother what her grandmother used to eat, and you'll be in good shape. Anything that was considered food 150 years ago is generally good for our bodies today.

THE GET YOUR GUT IN SHAPE
jump-start tips

1. **Drink pomegranate juice.** Pomegranates contain ellagic acid, which acts to protect against some metal toxicity by promoting its excretion. Always drink pomegranate juice with or after a protein to counterbalance the sugar it contains.

2. **Increase fiber intake.** Fiber not only promotes the removal of toxins excreted via bile from the liver, it also decreases the absorption of some toxins. Fiber-rich foods include green leafy vegetables such as spinach, kale, and lettuce; asparagus, carrots, zucchini, broccoli, cauliflower, cabbage, and Brussels sprouts; and fruits such as apples and berries.

3. **Stay hydrated.** The basic rule of drinking six to eight 8-ounce glasses a day still applies. If you want to get more specific, multiply your weight by 0.6 and that will give the amount of ounces you need in a day (if you're an athlete, multiply your weight by 0.75). Don't drink all your water at once—sip it throughout the day. Many ear, nose, and throat doctors say that drinking too much water at one time can produce postnasal drip and pharyngitis (inflammation of the part of the throat between the tonsils and the larynx). Plus studies have

shown that if you drink all those ounces of water all at once, you don't get the same benefit. It just goes right through you. Keep it on your desk. Keep it in your car. Keep it next to when you watch TV. Athletes have long known that water is important to keep up their energy levels and that performance is negatively affected by a lack of water. Studies have shown that a person who is as little as 2 percent dehydrated can experience up to a 10 percent decline in performance.

Another way to stay hydrated and energized is to eat fluid-filled foods, such as fresh fruits and vegetables. Skip dry packaged snacks such as pretzels in favor of apple wedges or celery stalks.

4. **Drink green tea.** Green tea contains plant-based nutrients called catechins, a type of flavonoid (potent antioxidants produced by plants to protect themselves from bacteria, parasites, and cell damage). In addition to being a cancer inhibitor, catechins have been shown to activate certain detoxification enzymes. Green tea has also been shown to promote "good" intestinal flora and PH balance and to support healthy bowel function, all of which aid the body's detox process. You don't have to drink huge amounts of green tea to get its benefits—one cup of tea contains between 100 to 200 mg of catechins, which is enough to account for approximately 90 percent of its beneficial effects. Don't forget that tea counts as your water intake, too. Try doing what they do in Asian countries—they take hot tea along with them wherever they go and sip it all day long.

5. **Take a sauna.** Saunas have been used around the world for centuries for detoxification and relaxation. A sauna (a small room or facility where people sit or recline in hot temperatures to sweat) rids your body of toxins and helps to improve overall circulation. To get the best effect, you should sit in a sauna for no more than 45 minutes. The object is to heat your fat cells sufficiently so that the toxins stored within them are released through your sweat glands.

6. **Begin an anti-inflammatory diet.** The good news is that inflammation can be reduced by choosing an anti-inflammatory diet.

Below is a list of inflammatory foods, which are to be avoided or chosen less often:

Chips
Corn
Cookies, cakes, etc.
Deep-fried foods

Fast foods
Gluten-containing products
Processed meats

The list that follows includes anti-inflammatory foods which are to be chosen more often:

Almonds
Apples
Avocados
Basil
Bell peppers
Black currants
Blueberries
Bok choy
Broccoli
Brussels sprouts
Cabbage
Cauliflower
Cayenne pepper
Chard
Chili peppers
Cinnamon
Cloves
Cod
Collards
Dark chocolate (at least 70% cacao*)
Extra virgin olive oil

Fennel
Flaxseed
Garlic
Green beans
Green onions
Green tea
Halibut
Hazelnuts
Herring
Kale
Kiwi
Leeks
Lemons
Limes
Mint
Mulberries
Olives
Oranges
Oregano
Papaya
Parsley
Pineapple (fresh)

Rainbow trout
Raspberries
Rhubarb
Rosemary
Salmon
Sardines
Snapper fish
Spinach
Strawberries
Striped bass
Sunflower seeds
Sweet potatoes
Thyme
Tomatoes
Tuna
Turmeric
Turnip greens
Walnuts
Whitefish

*Cacao is the bean that comes from the cacao tree. After it is processed (fermented and dried), it is referred to as cocoa, although the words are often used interchangeably.

Now that you've improved your eating habits and are on your way to having a healthy gastrointestinal system, are you still not feeling 100 percent? Is your energy still not where you'd like it to be? Every system in the body is influenced by every other system. If you make improvements in one area and you're still not seeing the results you'd like, you have to look at other systems as well. There are many factors at work that affect your digestive system besides the food you eat (or don't eat). If you're not getting enough rest, or if you are overstressed, your gut will not work properly. In the next chapter, you'll discover a variety of ways to improve your sleep habits and reduce the stress in your life.

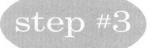

step #3

Improve Your Sleep and Reduce Your Stress

There have been several times in my life when I've had trouble sleeping. Because of that, I've learned a number of tricks to help me get to sleep. Perhaps the most important lesson is a motto I've learned to live by: *give sleep a chance.* I learned to condition my body to sleep. We're an impatient nation; we don't want to simply lie there and do nothing. But that may be just what we need to do. Cliché though it may be, try counting sheep, or shoes, or shamrocks—anything that gives you pleasure. Personally, I use numbers, counting backward from 100, and I do it over and over until I fall asleep. This process prevents me from thinking about what happened today or what might happen tomorrow.

Have you ever spent a restless night, unable to sleep, worrying about this, that, and the other until you finally drifted off, only to dream that you are driving a car with no brakes? Do you wake up in the morning feeling totally exhausted and unprepared to handle what you fear the day might bring? And then the next night, even though you're exhausted, are you still unable to get off the worry train?

That's what I call the sleep/stress continuum, when stress causes you sleepless nights and sleepless nights cause your stress to multiply. It happens to all of us, and if it happens to you more than just once in a while, it is one of the worst energy zappers you can encounter.

Don't you hate it when people say, "The solution is easy. Get more sleep and avoid stressful situations"? Okay. So I guess that means I have to quit my job, stop being a mother, steer clear of relationships, never get caught in traffic, and give up any other obligations I might be tempted to take on. In other words, stop living. Clearly, avoiding stress is impossible. Luckily, you can learn to reduce stress, or at least modify how you react to it. And you can learn to improve the quality and quantity of your sleep so that you have more energy to better cope with life's little surprises.

IMPROVE YOUR SLEEP HABITS

It's 3:00 in the afternoon. You're sitting at your desk. Your thoughts begin to get fuzzy. Your eyes begin to close. Your fingers, flying across the keyboard just a few minutes earlier, now seem too heavy to lift. You're nowhere near finished with the report that's due by the end of the day. And all you want to do is sleep.

Common sense will tell you that all the energy advice in the world won't help you if you're just not getting enough sleep. And the truth is that most of us are not getting the zzz's we need. Sleep deprivation is epidemic in our society. Animal studies have shown that this can be fatal, and it's no different for human beings. And there's now evidence that shows that how much sleep you get could be one of the most important factors influencing your energy production, your longevity, and even your weight.

In recent years, there have been a number of major studies showing that failing to get enough sleep heightens the risk for a variety of illnesses, including cancer, heart disease, diabetes, and obesity. People who are sleep deprived have high levels of inflammation. Sleep deprivation resets our internal clock, throwing off our endocrine, immune, and metabolic systems. Sleep enhances wellness by supporting adrenal-gland function, which in turn helps balance weight and emotions while reducing sugar cravings. If you're not averaging at least seven hours of sleep at night, you're putting your health at risk.

Sleep Statistics

It is estimated that 50 million to 70 million Americans suffer from a chronic sleep disorder. Women are twice as likely to suffer from insomnia than men. According to the National Center for Sleep Disorders Research at the National Institutes of Health, about 30 to 40 percent of adults say they have some symptoms of insomnia within a given year, and about 10 to 15 percent of adults say they have chronic insomnia. If you need more proof that trouble sleeping is a common experience, according to the National Sleep Foundation's 2009 *Sleep in America* poll, the odds that an adult has difficulty falling asleep at least a few nights a week are 1 in 3.45. And 1 in 6.25 adults have difficulty falling asleep every night or almost every night.

To find out if you're sleep deprived, answer the questions below:

❖ Does it take you longer than 15 minutes to fall asleep at night?

❖ Do you wake up during night?

❖ Do you need an alarm clock to wake up?

❖ Do you consistently get fewer than eight hours of sleep per night?

❖ Do you wake up groggy and moody instead of refreshed and alert?

❖ Are there days when you just can't get out of bed?

❖ Do you have times when you can't mentally focus?

❖ Is lethargy ruining your ability to work?

Fatigue can be a debilitating condition that results in "yes" answers to the questions above. It can also result in loss of appetite and stamina, and it can even contribute to low self-esteem. You may have experienced energy shifts that you've attributed to being too busy or just to getting older.

Sleep is essential for maintaining optimal health and strength. It is both restorative and rejuvenating for your body. It only takes a few nights without quality, deep sleep to leave you tired, confused, lethargic, and moody. When we don't get enough quality sleep, we look at the world through fog-covered glasses. On the other hand, restful sleep sets up the brain for high energy and a positive outlook.

ADRENAL GLANDS, CORTISOL, SLEEP, AND STRESS

Before I give you more suggestions to improve your sleep and reduce your stress, I think it's important that you understand a little of the biology that governs our stress responses and our ability to get a good night's sleep. When it comes to stress and sleep, a wide variety of factors can be involved, both external and internal.

Francine came to my office with what she thought was a hormone problem. "I think I'm premenopausal," she said. "I'm having such problems getting to sleep. I think I need hormone-replacement therapy." She had been my patient for almost a year, and I was sure that wasn't the problem. So I asked her if anything unusual had been going on in her life for the past several months and if she'd changed her routine in any way. The only thing she could think of, she said, was that she had been given a major project at work, and to relieve her stress, she went to the gym for an hour almost every day. The only time she could fit it into her schedule was at about 8:00 at night.

Fortunately for Francine, this was an easy fix. I did recommend a form of natural hormone therapy: I suggested she go to sleep earlier, wake up earlier, and go to the gym before work. That way would she have more energy for her project, and she wouldn't be stimulating her energy hormones right before bedtime. Francine took my advice and now goes to the gym at 6:00 A.M., is in bed by 10:00 P.M. every night, and sleeps like a baby. Hopefully by reading the next few pages, you'll understand why this simple switch in the timing of events can have such a dramatic effect.

External factors such as eating or exercising too late in the evening can be changed fairly easily. It takes a little more effort and possibly some changes in lifestyle to affect the internal factors. The most important internal factors usually originate from the adrenal glands and a particular hormone they produce called cortisol. It turns out that learning to change some of the externals of sleep and stress (diet, behavior, and environment) can have a profound impact on how well the internal factors function.

Adrenal glands are triangular-shaped endocrine glands that sit on top of the kidneys. At the center of each gland is a medulla, which is surrounded by the cortex. The medulla secretes epinephrine (adrenaline) and norepinephrine, two hormones that are involved in the fight-or-flight response, directly increasing the heart rate, causing energy stores to release glucose, and increasing blood flow to skeletal muscles. The cortex produces hormones (including cortisol) that regulate the body's metabolism, the balance of salt and water in the body, the immune system, and sexual function. The adrenal glands also release DHEA-S, a precursor of testosterone.

When the adrenal glands are not functioning optimally, you can have a condition that is known as adrenal fatigue. Adrenal fatigue often develops after periods of intense or lengthy physical or emotional stress, when overstimulation of the glands leave them unable to meet your body's needs.

Some of the symptoms of adrenal fatigue include:

❖ Excessive fatigue and exhaustion

❖ Waking up tired even though you get enough sleep

❖ Being overwhelmed by or unable to cope with stress

❖ Craving salty and sweet foods

❖ Feeling most energetic in the evening

❖ Having low stamina

❖ Slow to recover from injury, illness, or stress

❖ Difficulty concentrating, brain fog

❖ Poor digestion

❖ Consistent low blood pressure

❖ Extreme sensitivity to cold

The Cortisol Connection

One of the most important jobs of the adrenal glands is the production of cortisol, a hormone that is involved in a number of the body's functions. Among other things, cortisol:

❖ Regulates carbohydrate, fat, and protein metabolism

❖ Regulates blood pressure

❖ Converts amino acids to glucose (sugar)

❖ Promotes the release of insulin to maintain steady blood-sugar levels

❖ Promotes the breakdown of fats into fatty acids and glycerol

Cortisol's primary purpose is to break down body tissues to be used as an energy source. Cortisol is also known as "the stress hormone" because in times of stress, higher levels of cortisol are released into the body. That's when the fight-or-flight response begins—your heart begins to race, you have a sudden burst of energy, your blood pressure increases, and your senses seem suddenly sharper than they were a minute ago. If there's danger lurking, you need all the help you can get. You especially need a readily available supply of energy, and it is cortisol's job to make it accessible to you.

The release of cortisol is designed to be a short-term solution to fill an urgent need for energy. When this hormone level remains high for a sustained period of time, however, it can cause a variety of health problems. For instance, instead of sharpening your mind, prolonged elevated cortisol can result in impaired cognitive performance. During my residency program (which was back in the '80s) it was standard to be on call for a 36-hour shift. Sometimes you actually wouldn't sleep for 48 to 72 hours. If it was a busy night, you wouldn't get a moment to rest. I was constantly on edge. My brain and my body were running on adrenaline. Life-and-death situations were constant. Working that many hours has since been outlawed because too many critical mishaps occurred, too many misjudgments. Even though you were awake and active and it seemed as if you were on top of things, your brain wasn't working the way it was supposed to. The body is on an adrenaline rush during that period of time; however, the neurotransmitters and other hormones couldn't keep up and you became like a zombie. Elevated cortisol can also result in elevated blood-sugar levels, or hyperglycemia. Other negative consequences include decreased bone and muscle mass, a weakened immune system, increased abdominal fat, and, of course, insomnia.

Cortisol naturally spikes and dips within a 24-hour period. This is part of our natural circadian rhythm, an internal timekeeper that is associated with external cycles such as daylight, darkness, and changing seasons. A hormone called adrenocorticotropic hormone (ACTH), produced by the pituitary gland, communicates with the adrenal glands and tells them when to release cortisol. When you're sleeping, the release signal is virtually turned off. The signal is turned on again, usually between 7:00 A.M. and 8:00 A.M., and you get a strong surge of cortisol which keeps you going for most of the day. Then, late in the afternoon, cortisol levels spike again. When you go to bed, cortisol levels are decreasing, reaching their lowest point between midnight and 4:00 A.M. During this time, the body is recovering from the hard work of the day. If you're not sleeping properly, you disrupt cortisol's natural schedule, and your adrenal glands don't get the chance to recover. The release signal is stuck in the "on" position. It's like being on cocaine throughout the night; cortisol is a stimulant and it will keep you awake. When you do manage to get some sleep, your cortisol resources upon awakening are much less than they should be, and you remain tired throughout the day.

Cortisol and Low Blood Sugar

As have have mentioned, cortisol helps regulate blood-sugar levels. In Chapter 2, I suggested that instead of the usual three meals a day, we should be eating every three to four hours. One of the reasons for that is to maintain cortisol at its proper levels. Going too long between meals or snacks lowers blood-sugar levels. Low blood-sugar levels trigger the pituitary gland to release ACTH, which signals the release of cortisol, which in turn causes blood sugar levels to rise. When you continue a pattern of long time spans between meals, the adrenals end up working harder than they should to keep up with the body's demands. Another consequence of going too long between meals is that you then tend to consume high-sugar and-high carbohydrate meals, which overstimulate insulin production. Your blood sugar then swings crazily from high to low, which again triggers cortisol to be released.

At this point, your adrenal glands are going to go on strike. The pituitary "boss" has been yelling at them for days: "Speed up production. No, slow it down. No, shut it off. No, get back to work. More, more, we need more. No, wait, too much! Too much!" The adrenal glands don't have time to recover from being overworked, and they just can't function as efficiently as they should.

One of the most serious consequences of adrenal fatigue and low blood sugar is that it can keep you from getting a good night's sleep. When your blood sugar is lower than normal during the night, the pituitary alarm signal goes off and wakes you up so that you can refuel and replenish the sugar supply.

The good news is that if you follow the three-to-four hour rule and eat meals that contain quality proteins, fats, and complex carbohydrates, you won't experience those tremendous highs and lows of blood sugar levels, the adrenals will have time to recover, and cortisol production can get back to its natural rhythm. If you are having trouble sleeping through the night, a healthy snack before bedtime just might help. Try having a slice of whole-grain bread with almond butter or a few whole-grain crackers with cheese. It just may help you get the rest you need.

If you suspect that you have an adrenal or cortisol imbalance, talk to your health-care professional about having an adrenal stress index (ASI). This saliva test measures the production of several adrenal hormones, including cortisol and DHEA-S across a 24-hour period. You can read more about testing in Chapter 9.

Sleep and Growth Hormone

Another hormone that is important to sleep patterns is human growth hormone (HGH). An abundance of HGH is produced by the pituitary gland when we are very young. This growth hormone plays a significant role in energy production, muscle and tissue growth, brain function, bone strength, metabolic development, intracellular communication, and healing capacity. Growth hormone levels increase when we are asleep, reaching a peak during the first few hours. Production of growth hormone drops off dramatically in the body in our 30s and 40s, which may be a contributing factor to sleep disorders as we age. Conversely, if we don't get enough sleep, we don't release enough growth hormone to do the repair work necessary to keep us healthy and energized.

HOW TO GET MORE AND BETTER SLEEP

There are many reasons for not getting enough sleep. Some, as we just learned, are biological. Others are behavioral. Don't assume there's something wrong with you if you can't fall asleep right away. If you're having trouble sleeping, try some of these tips and see if they do the job:

- ❖ **Reserve the bedroom for sex and sleep.** You want your mind to register your bedroom as a place for only two activities: sleeping and making love. If your bedroom is also your workout room (do you have a treadmill in your bedroom?) or your workspace, it will be difficult to separate the two activities when it's time to go to bed. One of my patients, the daughter of a famous rock star who lived in a large bedroom suite on her father's estate, couldn't understand why she was having so much trouble getting to sleep. When I asked her to describe her bedroom activities, she told me that she had recently had a stripper pole installed in the room, and often entertained her friends there. She and her friends used the pole just for fun and exercise. She didn't realize that by doing so, she was associating her bedroom with a place to be active, not a place to relax and leave the day behind. She moved the pole to a downstairs family room and was soon back to enjoying a restful night's sleep.

❖ **Avoid alcohol, especially right before bedtime.** Although it can help you unwind, booze actually interrupts your natural sleep pattern, causing you to wake up about four hours after you go to sleep when you metabolize the alcohol and the sedating effect wears off.

❖ **Stop drinking all liquids two hours before bedtime.** Drinking any liquid will make you want to pee only a few hours into your sleep. And getting up once in the night to pee is one time too many.

❖ **Limit caffeine and sugar intake.** You may want to indulge during the day to help you stay awake, but you'll be defeating your purpose as these substances will destroy your circadian rhythm and keep you awake all night as well.

❖ **Avoid stimulating activities an hour before bedtime.** According to a 2008 National Sleep Foundation survey, many people who have trouble sleeping engage in stimulating activities an hour before getting into bed at least a few nights a week. They found that 43 percent of their respondents completed household chores such as vacuuming or washing dishes, 33 percent were on the computer or the Internet, and a whopping 90 percent watched TV (that may seem like passive activity, but not if you're watching violent programs or the evening news). Television isn't as relaxing as it may seem; after all, it's designed to keep you watching. That's why I have a no-television-in-the-bedroom policy, for my patients and for myself. I have a three-level home; all the bedrooms are on the third level, and there are no TVs allowed. My kids, however, have learned to get around this by downloading television shows onto their computers, so I now have to be extra vigilant to make sure all electronics are off well before bedtime.

❖ **If you can't sleep, get up.** Don't toss and turn for more than 20 to 30 minutes. Get out of bed and out of the room. Do something relaxing, such as listening to music or reading, in another part of the house until you feel sleepy, then return to the bedroom and try again. I have patients who get panic attacks every night before they have to go to bed because they think it's going to take them hours to get to sleep, and the idea of tossing and turning in bed for two hours causes extreme anxiety. That's why it's best to get up, do something relaxing, and go back to bed when you're ready to sleep.

❖ **Get some recovery sleep on the weekends.** What does it matter if you lose an hour or two of sleep here and there during the week? You can always sleep late on Saturday and Sunday, right? Not everyone agrees on the answer to that question, but a 2010 study published in the journal *Sleep* found that those few extra hours of "recovery sleep" are good for us and can actually undo some of the damage caused by sleep deprivation. For five straight nights, study participants were only allowed to sleep for four hours a night. The researchers then sampled their levels of alertness and neurobehaviors (the way the brain affects emotion, behavior, and learning) during the day. All of the participants suffered from fatigue and loss of motor and cognitive speed. On the sixth night, each participant was granted a period of recovery sleep that lasted about ten hours. The study's authors found that this extra sleep restored participant's neurobehaviors, including levels of alertness and their ability to concentrate. However, they also found that it took most participants more than one ten-hour night of sleep to fully recuperate.

❖ **Keep yourself in mind.** Women often take care of everyone else before they take care of themselves, which often means they're up early and into bed late. Take a step back and look at your lifestyle. Are there things you can change? Are you taking on unnecessary burdens that family members might be able to share? How much of what you're doing is truly essential and how much is just habit?

From Dr. Eva's Files

Kathleen O. came to me complaining that she was completely exhausted. I asked her to describe for me a typical day in her life. She said, "I get up at about 6:00 in the morning. I prepare breakfast and lunch for my sons. I take them to school. I get back home about 7:30 or 8:00, and then I go back to sleep for about two hours, before I have to get ready for my part-time job."

I asked, "Why are you going back to sleep?" She explained that she doesn't get to bed until well after midnight. I asked her why she didn't go to bed earlier, and she said she had to stay up to make sure her 16-year-old son went to sleep.

I thought it was a bit odd that her son couldn't take responsibility for his own bedtime. Kathleen told me that he was a swimmer, and he didn't get home until after 7:00 at night, at which point he had to have dinner, start his homework, and prepare for his SATs. He didn't have the discipline himself, so his mother (a single parent) felt she had to watch over him, including seeing that he got enough sleep. She knew that she was cheating herself out of the rest she needed, but her son was her priority. However, she didn't realize how much it was affecting her; what she thought was a medical problem turned out to be a time-management problem with her son. Her lack of sleep was clouding her judgment about what was best for herself and her sons.

A lot of women put their children first, but they don't realize that by doing so they can't function effectively—they take it out on their children or on themselves or on their spouse or on the people at work. They think they're doing the right thing by giving all of themselves to their children but they're really hurting themselves and everyone around them.

Together, Kathleen and I made a plan to give her sons more independence—they made their own school lunches and the 16-year-old got a car so he could drive himself and his brother to school—and to give her more time to get the restorative sleep she needed. Within just a few weeks, Kathleen was feeling much more energized and able to take better care of her family.

Can You Sleep and Breathe at the Same Time?

My friend Anna and I were out to dinner one night. Naturally, our conversation turned to the subject of our husbands. Anna confessed to me that she and her husband had been arguing lately. "About what?" I asked. Her face turned red, her neck got blotchy, and she could barely get the words out. I expected something terrible. "Apparently," she said, "I snore."

For some reason, women are usually terribly embarrassed to admit they snore. Perhaps we see it as a masculine trait (men do snore more than women). Snoring is nothing to be embarrassed about, but it can be a sign that you should be concerned about some of your sleep patterns.

Do people ever tell you that you snore like a buzz saw? Do you sleep for eight hours or more and still wake up tired? Has anyone ever heard you gasping in the middle of the night? Do you fall asleep sitting, reading, watching TV, or driving? Do you have chronic problems with memory or concentration? If you've answered yes to one or more of these questions, you might have sleep apnea. Obstructive sleep apnea (OSA) is a condition in which there are repeated interruptions of breathing during sleep that cause oxygen levels to drop. Sleep apnea causes you to wake up multiple times in the night so that you never get the rest you need, are tired during the day, and can't function up to par. People with untreated sleep apnea stop breathing repeatedly during their sleep, sometimes hundreds of times during the night and often for a minute or longer. When that happens, the body's defense mechanism kicks in and you wake up so that you can get the oxygen you need. This awakening is usually so brief that you don't even remember it. People with OSA often think they've slept very well through the night.

If you are a heavy snorer, you are at a much greater risk of having OSA, which is most often diagnosed in overweight men with a large neck circumference, although many women suffer from it as well. Sleep apnea has also been linked with several diseases including hypertension, diabetes, cardiovascular disease, congestive heart failure, and even sudden death. People with sleep apnea are also frequently prone to gastroesophageal reflux disease (GERD), a digestive disorder commonly known as heartburn that is caused by gastric acid flowing from the stomach into the esophagus. Sleep apnea, which occurs more frequently with advancing age, is very common and affects more than twelve million Americans, according to the National Institutes of Health.

Obstructive sleep apnea occurs when the muscles in the back of your throat relax and your airway narrows or closes as you breathe in. It is a very serious cause of fatigue, but luckily it is easily treatable.

First, you need to get a clear diagnosis of sleep apnea. This is often done in special sleep centers, where you spend the night hooked up to equipment that monitors your heart, lung, and brain activity, breathing patterns, arm and leg movements, and blood-oxygen levels. Or your doctor may provide you with a portable monitoring device, such as the SNAP machine we prescribe in our office, which can measure your heart rate, blood-oxygen level, airflow, and breathing patterns. The patient takes it and sleeps with it in the comfort of his or her own home, as opposed to a formal sleep-apnea test. If the results are abnormal, your doctor may prescribe a particular treatment, or may recommend that you go to a sleep center for further evaluation.

One of the most common treatments for sleep apnea is weight loss, and that's the first thing we suggest to people. An obese abdomen makes expanding the chest more difficult. It becomes harder to take a breath because the fat is being pushed up against the diaphragm.

If a patient can't lose the weight, she might be prescribed a continuous positive airways pressure (CPAP) machine, which delivers air pressure through a mask placed over your nose while you sleep. It works by keeping your upper airway passages open while you sleep. It is effective, but it is also cumbersome and some people find it too uncomfortable to use. There are other types of appliances that can be used, and a number of devices available from your dentist. It may take some trial and error to find the one that is right for you. For the most severe cases, there are surgical options as well.

Many of my patients tell me they want to try to make lifestyle changes before they try the CPAP or dental appliances. In that case, I recommend they:

❖ **Avoid alcohol and tranquilizers.** These relax the muscles in the back of the throat, which can interfere with your breathing. Overrelaxed breathing muscles lead to increased snoring and the increased possibility of breathing stoppage.

❖ **Stop smoking.** Yet another reason to quit the nasty habit! Smoking tends to create congestion in the upper air passages. Also, the chemicals in cigarettes irritate the respiratory system.

❖ **Try side sleeping.** Sleeping on your back can cause your tongue and soft palate to rest against the back of your throat and block your airway. Here's a good trick: if you start out sleeping on your side but find that you roll over onto your back in the middle of the night, attach a small rubber ball to the back of your pajama top or nightgown.

Sleep Aids

When I was going through my own bout of debilitating fatigue, I was hardly able to sleep at all. My sleep patterns were completely off. After being tested, I discovered I had deficiencies in magnesium as well as vitamins B_1, B_2, and B_{12}. I began taking supplements to fix the problem, but until they started to work, I needed help getting to sleep. I chose the prescription sleep aid Lunesta. It is not habit forming or addictive, and according to the FDA, it can be taken daily for up to a year with no consequences. In my opinion, you don't need to be a "hero" and deny yourself the ability to sleep until your body chemistry is back to normal. Many times, you get into an unhealthy cycle that prevents you from sleeping. If you can alter that pattern by taking a sleep aid, then your body will reset itself, at which point you can slowly taper off the sleep aid and sleep naturally again. If lifestyle changes and natural herbal remedies (as listed in the next section) don't work, I then recommend to my patients a short-term course of therapy with prescription sleep aids such as Sonata, Lunesta, or Ambien.

Vitamins and Herbal Sleep Remedies

There are a wide variety of vitamins and herbal supplements that are not as intensive as sleep aids, but that can—along with the sleep hygiene steps mentioned earlier—help you get a good night's sleep. Remember, because of the potential for side effects and interactions with medications, you should always consult a health-care professional before taking dietary supplements. Some of these supplements include:

❖ **Adrenal Complex:** Adrenal complex plays a crucial role in supporting the health of the adrenals. Ingredients include schizandra, which has traditionally been used in Chinese medicine, is regarded as an adaptogenic herb. Schizandra is used to bring balance to the adrenals and support a general sense of well-being. Also regarded as an adaptogenic herb, rhodiola has been used for centuries in Russia to help with fatigue and stress, and to boost immune health. Siberian ginseng is used to help boost energy levels, decrease fatigue, and improve overall immune health. Licorice root has a long history of use including adrenal support. Licorice root increases the half-life of endogenous cortisol.

❖ **Magnesium:** Magnesium is often called the anti-stress mineral because it has a calming effect on the nervous system when taken. Although some women experience the unpleasant side effect of loose stool, it actually helps the majority of my patients, most of whom complain about constipation. Foods that are high in magnesium include: alfalfa, apples, apricots, avocados, bananas, black-eyed peas, blackstrap molasses, brown rice, cantaloupe, capsicum, figs, garlic, grapefruit, green leafy vegetables, lemons, lima beans, nuts, parsley, peaches, and whole grains.

❖ **Inositol:** Inositol promotes overall relaxation and maintains the metabolism of serotonin. It is also used for promoting brain wellness and female hormone health through its role in supporting optimal liver function. It is a member of the B-complex family and has been used to treat anxiety and panic attacks.

❖ **B vitamins:** Insomnia can be caused by deficiencies in the B vitamins, so it may be helpful to consume foods that are good sources of B_6 (egg yolks, grains, seeds, and yeast), B_{12} (walnuts, bananas, tuna, peanuts, and sunflower seeds), and B_5 (also known as pantothenic acid, can be found in fish and milk).

❖ **5-HTP:** 5-HTP is a naturally occurring amino acid, and is the immediate precursor to serotonin, the brain nutrient for relaxation. A Norwegian study showed that 5-HTP can affect sleep patterns by increasing the levels of serotonin, which is needed for sleep. Serotonin is needed to produce melatonin, the hormone that regulates sleep-wake cycles. Studies have also shown that 5-HTP may improve the quality of sleep by lengthening the REM stage (a mentally active period in which dreaming and rapid eye movements take place) and deep non-REM sleep without increasing total sleep time by raising serotonin levels.

❖ **Tryptophan:** Tryptophan is well known as one of the reasons everyone falls asleep after a big Thanksgiving feast, as turkey is an excellent source. Tryptophan is also an amino acid, and its main function is to manufacture serotonin. It is available in supplements or in foods such as avocados, milk, cottage cheese, nuts, bananas, lean meat, tuna, shellfish, and of course, turkey.

❖ **Melatonin:** Although this is one of the best-known sleep supplements, it's not one of my favorites. Melatonin is a hormone secreted by the pineal gland in the brain. It helps regulate other hormones and maintains the body's circadian rhythm (which is why it has a reputation for being good for reducing jet lag). When the lights go out, melatonin production begins. However, if you get up at night to go to the bathroom and turn on the light, you turn off the melatonin trigger, which may be why it's often so hard to get back to sleep.

I don't recommend melatonin for several reasons. First, since melatonin is a hormone, it can affect many internal body processes. Second, there is actually little evidence that taking melatonin supplements will help you fall asleep significantly faster or help you stay asleep longer. And it seems that this supplement only works for sleep problems if your melatonin levels are low, which means it may work best if you are elderly, because melatonin levels drop off as you age. If you choose to take melatonin supplements, side effects may include daytime sleepiness, dizziness, headaches, abdominal discomfort, confusion, sleepwalking, and nightmares.

Melatonin may also interact with various medications, including:

- Anticoagulants (blood-thinning medications)
- Immunosuppressants (drugs that lower the body's normal immune response, for instance, medications taken following a transplant to prevent rejection)
- Diabetes medications
- Birth-control pills

My strongest argument against melatonin is for menstruating women. Melatonin can affect prolactin, which is the hormone that stimulates the mammary glands to produce breast milk. Prolactin can actually effect the thyroid, as well as estrogen and progesterone production, which is why I'm not a fan for women who are menstruating. I don't have as much of a concern about it for women who are already menopausal.

Some studies have shown that taking melatonin for longer than two months may be harmful, and there is no consensus as to the best dose of melatonin. If you do take melatonin, make sure the supplements are made of artificial ingredients, rather than from animals. Melatonin from animals can contain viruses or other contaminants.

REDUCE YOUR STRESS

Is it difficult for you to calm down and relax?
Are you tense and irritated most of the time? Argumentative?
Are you experiencing indigestion, diarrhea, or constipation?
Has your appetite recently decreased?
Do you have trouble sleeping?
Are you experiencing nightmares?
Do you often feel achy all over, especially in the back, neck, and shoulders?
Do you notice a rapid or erratic pulse? Anxiety attacks?
Have there been sudden changes in your weight?
Has there been a decrease in your libido?

Answering "yes" to any of these questions could mean that you are undergoing stress. Technically, stress is a disruption of homeostasis, which is the ability to maintain a stable condition. Under those terms, stress, which we usually think of as a negative, can apply to positive events as well, for example wonderful surprises, passion, or an artistic or athletic competition. Stress is anything that upsets your equilibrium, whether it's good or bad.

Stress is, in many cases, subjective. What one person finds stressful may be stimulating to another. I love to ski at a high speed down a mountainside; for me it is the ultimate thrill. For you, it may be something to be avoided at all costs. There is "good" stress and "bad" stress. Good stress generally refers to short-lived experiences that a person can master and come away with a sense of exhilaration and accomplishment (acing an exam, riding a roller coaster). Some people thrive on the energy and adrenaline rush they get from stress; it gives them a feeling of being on the edge and at the top of their game. Bad stress experiences are often prolonged or recurrent, emotionally draining, and physiologically exhausting or dangerous (caring for someone with a chronic illness, being laid off from a long-time job). There is no sense of mastery or control. This kind of stress can easily become distress, which can be destructive to mind and body.

Whatever it is that stresses you out causes a very particular physiological reaction, one that was developed as part of our evolutionary survival skills. It's that now familiar fight-or-flight response, an ancient genetic pathway that taught us to fear and run from saber-toothed tigers and cave bears. Genetically, we're stone-agers living in the 21st-century world. Cave bears have been replaced by the 24/7 work ethic, too many things to do every day, and no time to relax or to get enough sleep. Even stress itself has become more complicated than ever before. We may not be threatened by wild animals on a daily basis, but, because we are inundated every moment with instantaneous news reports from around the world, we now worry not only about our own survival and the survival of our families, but also about the survival of the planet.

Normally, if you faced a stressful situation, your body would go into danger mode and then return to normal once the threat had passed. But your body cannot tell the difference between the threat of a wild animal and the threat of a looming deadline. The stress response is the same in both situations. So what happens when you face the kind of modern stress that follows us all day and well into the night? Often, the body will run out of energy reserves and simply exhaust itself.

Sources of Chronic Stress*			
Mental and Emotional	Tissue Damage/ Inflammation/ Pain	Glycemic Dysregulation	Others
Anger	Surgery	Skipping meals	Sleep deprivation
Worry	Trauma	High carbohydrate intake	Temperature extremes
Fear	Injury	Low-calorie diets	Excessive exercise
Grief	Infections	Alcoholism	Chronic illness
Bitterness	Inhalant allergies	Nutritional deficiencies	Noise pollution
Hopelessness	Food sensitivities		Caffeine or drug abuse
Guilt	Crohn's disease		
Depression	Colitis		
Anxiety	Celiac disease		
Job/ performance demands	Arthritis		
Financial pressures	Toxins: heavy metals, molds, chemicals		
Relationship conflicts			

*Used with permission from *Physician Road Map: Interpretive Guide and Suggested Protocols for the A.R.K. Adrenal Stress Profile,* Ortho Molecular Products.

The Adrenal Glands Back in Action

Stress begins in your brain. Whether there's something "out there" that can be perceived as dangerous (as in a brush fire very near your house) or exciting (as in your first motorcycle ride), your brain picks up the vibe and sends a signal to the adrenal gland to release the hormone adrenaline. That triggers the release of glucose into your blood, ramps up your heartbeat, and raises your blood pressure (among other things). At the same time, the hypothalamus (the hormonal regulation center) sends a signal to the pituitary gland, which stimulates the adrenal cortex to produce cortisol.

So now you have adrenaline and cortisol running around your brain, trying to help you cope with a life-threatening situation—even though in reality you may be trying to cope with a computer that crashes and destroys your expense report. And these stress hormones can linger in your system long after the stressful situation is over. If the brain is overloaded with stress hormones, it can literally excite cells to death. That is why it is so important to learn ways to cope with the stresses in our lives, small or large, real or perceived, so that we don't get to the point of chronic fatigue and overwhelming exhaustion.

De-stress Versus Distress: Finding Ways to Relieve Stress

The degree to which we experience stress is different for everyone. And the same person can react to stress in different ways at different times. You may be cool as a cucumber even though your boss is screaming at you for something that wasn't your fault, yet fall to pieces if your child suffers a bloody nose. Stress is a natural part of life. In fact, the stress response (the fight-or-flight reaction and its physiological changes mentioned earlier) is present in all species, in all cultures, and in all individuals. You can't make stress disappear but you can learn ways to find relief from its potentially harmful consequences.

Stress relief is one of the most important factors for living a long, productive, healthy life. Stress can cause or exacerbate obesity, inflammation, high blood pressure and reduced blood flow, allergies and sensitivities to environmental toxins, cognitive lapses, and sleep problems. It can cause or exacerbate symptoms such as headaches, neck aches, back pain, upset stomach, increased heart rate, poor circulation, sexual dysfunction, levels of panic/anxiety, depression, and some forms of arthritis. Stress can also damage your general health, your immune system, your skin, your weight, your levels of performance, and your energy levels.

Simply put, stress can make you old before your time. A 2004 study conducted in San Francisco looked deep into the DNA of stressed-out mothers of chronically ill children. They were looking at the mothers' telomeres, the "tip" of a strand of DNA, which protects the DNA from damage. Telomeres naturally get shorter as we age, until eventually the cell dies. That's one reason we lose eyesight, hearing, and muscle strength as we age. The 2004 study showed that stress has a similar effect, shortening the telomeres of the stressed-out moms, and aging them before their time. Women with the highest levels of perceived stress had telomeres shorter on average by the equivalent of at least one decade of additional aging compared to low-stress women. The good news is that those mothers who were better able to deal with stress—who had found ways of coping and maintaining a positive attitude—didn't suffer the same damage to their telomeres.

Telomeres get shorter as we age, but that can be accelerated by the way we live our lives—stress, drugs, lack of exercise, etc. accelerate the demise of the telomere. There is a genetic predisposition as to how quickly your telomeres shorten, but we're now finding that things such as growth hormone, estrogen, testosterone, and antioxidants can slow the rate of shortening. You do not have to continue to let stress strain your health and your energy supply. While you may not always be able to reduce the amount of stress you are under, there are numerous tools available to keep it in check:

❖ **Use music to reduce stress.** A study done at the University of Maryland Medical Center has shown that music is an excellent tool for reducing stress, whether you are playing an instrument or simply listening to the radio. Music releases neurotransmitters from the brain that relax the inner lining of the blood vessels, which increases blood flow and steadies the heart rate. It also calms your mental state by stimulating the release of endorphins, "feel good" hormones in the brain that help you feel happy and content. I used to get angry with my daughter when she would do her homework with hip hop music in the background, although I didn't mind if she was listening to classical music. However, the study showed that it doesn't matter what type of music it is—rock and roll, hip hop, or country work just as well as ballads or classical—as long as you vary the selections. Listening to the same song over and over again reduces the calming effect.

❖ **Take up meditation.** Meditation is a way to get "out of yourself," to try to quiet the mind and get beyond the "thinking" mind into a deeper state of relaxation or awareness. This can be achieved in many ways. You can begin by sitting upright with a straight spine, either cross-legged or on a firm chair with both feet on the floor, closing your eyes, and focusing on your breathing. Transcendental meditation involves the use of a mantra, a word or phrase or series of sounds that is chanted or sung as an incantation or prayer. You simply repeat the mantra silently over and over, and let your thoughts come and go as they will. This can be an effective mood elevator for many people. One of the reasons meditation works for relaxation is that it redirects the brain from worrying and disrupts the stress response.

❖ **Treat yourself to a massage.** Another way to disrupt the stress response is to get a massage. In fact, some studies have shown that massage therapy actually decreases cortisol levels. There are many types of massage available. Some of the more familiar include Swedish, Thai, deep tissue, hot stone, and Shiatsu.

Massage is one of the oldest, simplest forms of therapy and is a system of stroking, pressing, and kneading different areas of the body to relieve pain and relax, stimulate, and tone the body. There are studies that indicate that massage is critical for people under tremendous stress for decreasing anxiety and calming respiratory rates. Premature babies and infants who are massaged gained more weight and fared better than children who were not. It also has well-documented effects on immune-system performance. Research has shown that office workers who get massages regularly are more alert and perform better than people who don't. Massage has been shown to reduce the heart rate, lower blood pressure, relax muscles, improve range of motion, decrease anxiety, and increase endorphins (which is why you feel so good afterward). When I was in eastern Asia, one form of massage I saw everywhere was the foot massage. The people there feel that a lot of fatigue comes from the feet, one of the most important parts of the body. You would put your feet in very hot water, then they would begin pulling and rubbing your feet with oils and snapping your toes in a treatment that would last about an hour and a half. Even though they work only on your feet, you feel amazing when it's done.

❖ **Loosen up with Lipomassage.** Lipomassage is a deep tissue massage that was initially designed for smoothing cellulite and taking inches off of the body. The lipomassage machine uses rollers and gentle suctioning to deep massage the affected areas and increase circulation. It stimulates the fat cells and certain neurological receptors to trigger release of the trapped fat as far down as the third layer of skin. It also stimulates connective tissue to assist the body in restoring the texture of the skin; it disorganizes the fat clusters and stretches the connective tissue to smooth the dimpling skin. After a lipomassage session, you will likely feel an increase in energy and an overall feeling of relaxation. I personally use lipomassage not only to stay thin and energized, but because of all the skiing that I do on the weekends. Come Monday morning, the first thing I do is get my lipomassage because it's the most detoxifying deep tissue general massage I have ever experienced.

❖ **Relax with acupuncture.** It may seem like an oxymoron to relax while someone is sticking needles into your skin, but that is just what's been happening for the 5,000 years this ancient Chinese art has been around. As my husband learned on the Yangtze, acupuncture stimulates the body's ability to heal itself. Because traditional Chinese medicine is holistic, it treats the entire person— it addresses mental, physical, and emotional complaints. Traditional Chinese medicine views the human body as a highly complex electrical circuit. Like any electrical circuit, it must be kept in good working order if it is to function effectively, and if the circuit breaks down the result is illness. These breakdowns lead to blockage in the flow of chi (pronounced "chee," meaning vital energy) along pathways known as meridians, and inserting the acupuncture needles allows the chi to flow smoothly again. In Western medicine's view, it is thought that acupuncture primarily produces its effects through regulating the nervous system, helping the body to release endorphins and other neurotransmitters and neurohormones. These affect the parts of the central nervous system related to sensation and involuntary body functions, such as immune reactions and processes that regulate a person's blood pressure, blood flow, and body temperature. The World Health Organization has identified more than 40 ailments that are successfully treated with acupuncture, including eczema, headaches, PMS, immune system disorders, back pain, constipation, irritable bowel syndrome, anxiety, depression, insomnia, and stress.

❖ **Visit a chiropractor.** Chiropractic is about restoring function and stability of the spine. By releasing tension in the spine, muscles can be relaxed thereby relieving the pain associated with a back or neck problem. The purpose of chiropractic manipulation is to reduce stress and restore damaged nerve pathways, trying to get your brain to "talk" to every part of your body, to help you reach your full potential. The term *chiropractic* literally means "through the hands," and this is probably its most important function, according to Los Angeles chiropractor Shelly Bosten. "One of the reasons chiropractic is so important," says Bosten, "is because it is hands on. We all need to have that human touch by someone we trust." Part of her job, she says, is to form trusting relationships with her patients. "You've got to learn to trust the appropriate people," she says. "When you don't, your brain is constantly overstimulated, and you're not able to relax or have peace within your body because you don't have that trust. Your adrenal glands and entire endocrine system get overworked, and your body tightens up, which creates interference with your nervous and circulatory systems. Your body cannot function properly unless it is relaxed."

❖ **Invigorate through aromatherapy.** Aromatherapy uses concentrated essential oils of various plants for therapeutic purposes, particularly for the relief of pain, stress, nausea, and anxiety. You can add a few drops of essential oils to a bath or on a cold light bulb ring (a special ceramic or metal ring designed to be place directly on light bulbs). You can buy aromatherapy diffusers, which will disperse a fine mist of scent throughout a room, or you can add a few drops to a spray bottle filled with water and make your own diffuser. Although there are many essential oils that can be used to help you relax or make it easier to get to sleep, there are a few that are particularly good in fulfilling those needs, including lavender, chamomile, bergamot, sandalwood, and lemon. If you're looking for scents to help get more energized, try eucalyptus, peppermint, rosemary, jasmine, or cinnamon.

STRESSED-OUT EATING

When you're talking about stress, you're always confronted by a chicken-and-egg debate as far as eating is concerned: stress influences the food you eat, and the food you eat influences stress. You might experience an increase in appetite when you're stressed out. If so, you may be suffering from hyperglycemia, or high blood sugar. Your cortisol levels may be high. Essentially, the body is accessing and burning the fuel available in the food that's being eaten, rather than properly accessing stored fat. When that happens, you try to keep yourself energized by eating sugar and carbs.

On the other hand, stress may cause you to eat less often, but with larger meals. That might be a sign that stress is making your thyroid and adrenal glands sluggish and slowing down your metabolic activity. So you may also look to sugar and even caffeine to keep yourself going.

Whatever your reaction, the stress and stress-based eating cause disturbances in the hormone cholecystokinin (CCK), the substance that signals the brain to make you feel full. When you're under stress, you tend to eat faster; therefore, you don't give CCK enough time to send its signals to the brain. Stress often triggers the eating of comfort foods—foods high in fats and/or carbohydrates. You gobble down your foods in just a few minutes. Your stoplight system is out of order, and you eat until you go way past the point of feeling satisfied and well into being stuffed.

Carbohydrates also raise the level of serotonin in the body. Normally that's a good thing, because serotonin makes us feel good and helps us cope with stress. But because they make us feel good, many people learn to overeat carbohydrates (particularly snack foods, such as potato chips or pastries, which are rich in carbohydrates and fats) to make themselves feel better. Unfortunately, this overconsumption can also make us fat, which causes us stress, which causes us to overeat . . . Thus, the chicken-and-egg debate. By following the meal plans in Appendix I, you can balance the ratio of proteins, carbs, and fats, which will help keep serotonin production at healthy levels.

Getting to the Root of the Problem

Here's another chicken-and-egg situation: many woman who are under constant stress find that they are losing their hair. Stress can cause hair loss—and then the concern and embarrassment of hair loss can cause more stress! Many doctors ignore this complaint from their women patients, as they don't see it as life threatening. It may not be a life-or-death situation, but most women are horrified at the possibility of losing their hair. Many women worry more about losing their hair than they do about gaining weight, developing wrinkles, or needing a boob job or a face-lift. They are depressed because the quality and quantity of their hair isn't what it used to be. One way to help stop the loss is to take folic acid, which helps your body build keratin, a protein of which hair is made. You might want to check your health-food store for a combination supplement that contains 100 percent of your daily values of folic acid, zinc, biotin, and iron—all progrowth nutrients. However, the number one change you can make is to increase your protein intake. And never skip breakfast. Morning is when your energy is lowest, and your hair needs energy to grow. Watch your stress levels as well. Try some of the previously listed suggestions to relieve stress, which slows your digestive system and stops your hair follicles from getting the nutrients they need.

Hair growth and hair loss are complicated matters. If you're concerned about your hair, speak to a health-care professional as it could be an indication of any number of underlying health issues.

Herbal Stress Relievers

As with sleep aids, there are a wide variety of vitamins and herbal supplements that can help with stress relief. Some of these supplements include:

- ❖ **Ashwaganda:** This substance has traditionally been used in Ayurvedic medicine (the ancient Hindu science of health and medicine) and has been found to have antioxidant, antistress, and rejuvenating properties. It is said to promote calmness and satisfaction.

- ❖ **L-theanine:** This is an amino acid found in tea. It has been found to increase dopamine and serotonin production in the brain. It is also responsible for increasing alpha-brain wave activity, a sign of relaxation. L-theanine also influences the satiety signals coming from the brain, which means that the more tea you drink, the stronger the message to your brain that says, "I'm not hungry." This can help stop you from snacking on so many harmful carbohydrates.

- ❖ **Rhodiola:** This is an herb long used in traditional medicine in Russia and some Eastern European and Asian countries. Rhodiola is considered an adaptogen, a class of herbs said to help the body build resistance to stress. This supplement is customarily used to stimulate the nervous system, decrease depression, enhance work performance, and eliminate fatigue. Rhodiola may help fight fatigue and, in turn, boost mental performance in people struggling with stress-induced burnout.

- ❖ **Licorice root:** Licorice root supports the adrenal glands and helps to block the breakdown of cortisol, making it more available to the body. It also contains many antidepressant compounds and has the ability to improve resistance to stress. It can be very helpful when taken during times of both physical and emotional stress, after surgery or during convalescence, or when feeling tired and run down.

It's important to realize that no matter which supplements or methods you use to unwind and destress, the most important thing is to find time for yourself. Sometimes you just need to shut everything off, draw the curtains, turn off the phone, close down the computer, and relax, whether you're running a multimillion-dollar company or running after a three-year-old. It's important to find a quiet space of your own to sort out your thoughts and let your mind drift wherever it wants to go. You might try some deep breathing exercises as well: Inhale through the nose slowly and deeply to the count of ten. Exhale through the nose, slowly to the count of ten. Concentrating on the breathing and the counting can help quiet the mind and ease muscle tension. Repeat this exercise five times, anytime you feel stressed. As author Elisabeth Kubler-Ross once said, "There is no need to go to India or anywhere else to find peace. You will find that deep place of silence right in your room, your garden, or even your bathtub."

THE SLEEP AND STRESS
jump-start tips

1. **Set a gym curfew.** Try to work out before 4:00 P.M. Any later and you'll be revving up your body with adrenaline, which stimulates you and will keep you awake.

2. **Keep your bedroom cool.** It may seem like a good idea to keep the bedroom cozy and warm, but in reality a lower temperature helps your brain and body cool down for a good night's rest. It's like your computer going into sleep mode; it is conserving energy so that it is available when needed. Studies have shown that insomnia is associated with higher core-body temperatures, especially for older women.

3. **Establish a bedtime routine.** Go to bed at night and get up in the morning at the same time every day, even on weekends and holidays. Try giving yourself a little ritual to follow every night. That's what helps kids fall asleep—they get a story and a kiss every night. It's comforting, and it signals the body that it's time for sleep. Your ritual might be a warm bath or some soothing music or some nonstimulating reading just before bedtime.

4. **Sleep in complete darkness.** A study published in the Proceedings of the National Academy of Sciences in 2010 found that not only does complete darkness help you sleep, it helps prevent weight gain and depression. Mice exposed to light that was equivalent to leaving on a television, computer, or adjacent bathroom light gained 50 percent more weight than mice in total darkness. And hamsters subjected to nighttime light experienced a rise in depressive behaviors. The darker you can get your bedroom, the better. Even the small amount of light emitted by a nightlight can disrupt patterns of the adrenal gland and REM sleep, so be sure you have lightproof window curtains and/or use a sleep mask nightly.

5. **Try a little yoga.** Yoga, the ancient Indian art that is more than 5,000 years old, began as a way to attain spiritual enlightenment through physical and mental training. Today, there are many different forms of yoga practiced all over the United States. Yoga is great for toning and stretching the muscles at the same time that it relaxes the mind. It has been found to be beneficial for numerous conditions in which stress is a factor, such as headaches, asthma, high blood pressure, and anxiety, and it can have a healthful effect on the adrenal glands. One reason yoga has a calming effect may be that, as a 2007 study showed, an hour of yoga produced a surge of GABA, the neurotransmitter that helps produce a calm, focused state. And one of the best things about yoga is that it's good for everyone, no matter your age or shape.

There are several yoga *asanas,* that are referred to as postures and easeful stretches and not exercise, since exercise connotes a degree of strain. As Nirmala Heriza, certified yoga and clinical acupressure therapist says in her book, *Dr. Yoga: A Complete Guide to the Medical Benefits of Yoga,* "one of the primary reasons traditional Hatha Yoga is so effective for the adrenals and managing cortisol, is the absence of strain in the application and execution of the poses. Additionally, traditional Hatha Yoga incorporates a deep relaxation component essential to the overall effect of stabilizing and strengthening the cardiovascular and immune systems and balancing the endocrine system." Several of the yoga asanas Heriza recommends are:

♦   **Skull Shining:** Exhale completely through your nose. Inhale and produce a quick contraction of your abdomen, expelling the air. Then inhale and expel the air again. Repeat rapidly seven or eight times. Rest for a moment and begin a second round. Repeat three times. As you continue your practice, increase your capacity. Skull shining improves digestion, removes phlegm, and helps in the prevention and treatment of asthma and other respiratory diseases. It exhilarates blood circulation and energizes the entire body quickly. It can also help in the treatment of depression.

♦   **Alternate Nostril Breathing:** Sit in a comfortable cross-legged position. Make a loose fist with your right hand. Release your thumb and last two fingers. Relax your right arm against your chest and close your right nostril with your right thumb. Slowly exhale as much air as possible without strain through your left nostril. Then inhale through your left nostril and close it with the last two fingers of your right hand. Exhale through your right nostril. Upon inhalation, be sure to expand your stomach to full capacity to allow as much air as possible to enter your lungs. Upon exhalation, completely empty your lungs. Alternate your breathing this way a few times for as long as is comfortable. Then have a final exhalation through your right nostril and let your breath return to normal. Sit for a moment and observe the peaceful and calming effect of this practice on your system.

- **Full Forward Bend:** Lie on your back. Stretch your arms over your head. If you can do so comfortably, lock your thumbs. Slowly raise your arms, head, and chest, sitting up to an upright position. If you find this too difficult, just sit up comfortably, then raise your arms above your head. Slowly bend forward over your legs as far as you can comfortably go. Grasp your legs wherever you can reach comfortably—your ankles, calves, or thighs. Relax your face into your knees if you are able. Otherwise, relax your head to your chest. Relax in this position, breathing normally for ten seconds. Do not bend your knees. When coming out of this pose, lock your thumbs and stretch out over your legs, then rise to an upright position. Bring your hands to your lap and lie back comfortably in a supine position. The full forward bend pose affects the nervous system, promotes circulation through the coronary arteries, and relaxes the lining of the arterial walls, which can help to reduce plaque. In doing so, it reduces stress affecting the adrenals.

- **Half Locust:** Lie face down with your chin on the floor. Tuck your arms beneath your body, palms up, beneath your thighs. Do not bend your elbows. Keep your toes pointed. Raise your right leg without bending the knee. Allow all your weight to rest on your chest and arms. Slowly lower the leg. Relax. Do the same with the left leg. Turn your head to the side and rest. Keep your arms in place and return your chin to the floor. Repeat. Perform twice with each leg. This pose affects sympathetic nerve activity, slowing it down, helping to support adrenal function and to stabilize diastolic blood pressure.

6. **Practice prayer.** Whatever your religious or spiritual beliefs, one way to cope with a stressful situation is through prayer. Prayer isn't necessarily about religion. Prayer can be in the form of camping out and feeling one with nature. It doesn't really matter what you "pray" about, who you pray to, or where you do it.

I have my own form of prayer. My family and I have a vacation home that is a six-hour drive (if there's no traffic) from our home in Los Angeles. Many times I will drive up without my husband and ski by myself. People ask me all the time why I do it. For me, the few minutes I would spend on the chair lift would be my time of meditation and prayer. That's when I found my peace. Many people find that prayer helps them to get through their tough times by feeling that they have a higher power to lean on. I recently had a patient who told me that the only time she felt her stress melt away was when she went to church on Sundays because of the feeling of community it gave her and the energy she absorbed from being surrounded by a congregation full of people she cared about and who cared about her. She also said that it gave her comfort because she could walk into a church of her faith that might be thousands of miles from her home and still feel that there was a common goal and a common respect among the congregants even if they were of different ethnicities and didn't speak the same language. She could still feel at home and feel uplifted by the experience. Praying by yourself is a calming factor, she told me, while praying with others is an energy factor.

7. **Rely on your furry friends.** Your cat or dog may not come immediately to mind when thinking about stress relief, but studies have shown that people actually experienced less

stress when their pets were with them than when a supportive friend or even their spouse was present! Unless you truly hate animals, it's extremely difficult to stay in a bad mood when playing with a beloved pet. Of course, pets come with responsibilities—for some people that can mean added stress in their lives. For most people, however, the benefits of having a pet outweigh the drawbacks. Having a furry best friend can reduce stress in your life and bring you support when times get tough, which may be due to the fact that pets don't judge us—they just love us unconditionally.

No one lives a stress-free life, but following the tips in this chapter can help you cope with whatever challenges life presents. There's one challenge in life that doesn't often get discussed as a source of stress: maintaining your sexual desire and energy. I see a lot women who become stressed at the mere mention of having to have sex with their partners. Many women find that as they get older, sex becomes less and less of a priority. This in and of itself becomes a source of stress because they wonder if something is wrong with them, and because it takes a toll on their relationships. Sex becomes more about stress and less about relief. The libido seems to be fading, and sexual energy becomes difficult to find. This is not inevitable. There are a number of different steps you can take to help you get back into your sexual groove and enjoy that part of your life once again, as you will find out in Chapter 5 (probably the most popular chapter of this book).

step #4

Supercharge
Your Sexuality

Rachel is a beautiful 38-year-old working mother who loves her husband very much, yet fears she may have lost her capacity for sexual arousal and response. "Now that I finally know what turns me on and I feel confident about asking for what I want in bed, I have zero interest in sex," she confided. "I'm getting so depressed because now that the sexual spark has faded, I feel like the only thing that's holding my husband and me together is our two children. It's difficult for me to get out of bed in the morning for any reason other than to feed and clothe my children. I'm exhausted. I feel like part of my life is over. What is wrong with me?"

First, let me say that there's nothing seriously wrong with Rachel. Unfortunately, she represents millions of women who feel just the way she does. Second, she's in love with her husband and still finds him attractive, so he's not the problem. It's just that her libido is running out of steam. She's suffering from a sexual energy crisis.

Many women are tired and stressed out and feel guilty or depressed because of the sexual estrangement they feel from their partners. They have no energy for their daily obligations of caring for their children, getting their work done, and seeing to the household chores. For many, sex falls under this last category.

One thing I always tell my patients: Want good energy? Have good sex.

But having good sex is not always as easy as it sounds. Think about it. If you're like most women in this country, you have to cook meals, clean the house, and do the laundry. If you have children, you have to drive the kids to all their after-school activities and play dates. You have to socialize with your friends, your partner's friends, and the parents of your children's friends. Not to mention that you may have a career of your own to boot. It's no wonder you're burned out at the end of the day and would prefer to pick up a good book rather than pick up the love affair with your mate.

I can't tell you the number of patients I see who confide in me that they try to find any excuse to avoid intimacy with their partners. They brace themselves, knowing that if their partner is still awake by the time they get into the bedroom they will be expected to have sex. And they are so fearful of that, they will occupy themselves with anything they can find to put off entering that bedroom for as long as possible.

"Honey, I'll be up in a minute, I just have to prepare the kids' lunches for the morning."

"Honey, I'll be up in a minute, I just have to clean up the kitchen."

"Honey, I'll be up in a minute, I've just got to pay these bills."

"Honey, I'll be up in a minute, I (insert your favorite excuse here)."

Oftentimes, a woman is happiest when she finally does go to the bedroom only to find her mate snoring away. Let's be honest. She's relieved that she doesn't have to perform. Again, not because she doesn't love her partner, but because she simply has no energy left at the end of the day.

Women come to me from all over the world for help with their libidos, hormones, and sexual functioning. Some sexual problems can be due to medical (mostly hormonal) issues, and some may be due to lifestyle issues (too many demands, too little time). But no matter what the problem is, I tell them what I am telling you now—it really is possible to reenergize your sex life, reignite your libido, and reclaim deep sexual fulfillment.

The truth is that not much is known about why women experience a loss of libido. There is not much research on the subject. However, according to a 2009 article in *The New York Times,* around 30 percent of women between the ages of 20 and 60 go through extended periods where they have very little desire for sex—or would rather not have sex at all.

Hopefully, you've read the previous chapters and have begun to reclaim your personal energy by working on your eating habits and your sleep hygiene. Now it's time to revitalize your sexual energy. As you read this chapter, you will learn not only how modern medicine can help you, but also how ancient Eastern philosophies and techniques may help you get your sex life back. You'll learn how a few simple lifestyle changes can get you feeling revitalized and sexually healthy again. You'll find out how to light up your pleasure centers (including your brain, the body's largest erogenous zone), and as a result, you will have more energy for your love relationship.

But, if you're feeling inspired to light a fire under your cold sex life, there are seven easy steps you can take in the Jump-Start box at the end of the chapter. If you want to get started on it immediately, turn to page 155, then come back and read the rest of the chapter. I guarantee the Jump Starters will get you back in the mood and finally have you saying, "Honey, I'll be up in a minute—and I hope you are, too!"

Sex and the Rock Star

Perla Hudson has been with her husband for more than a decade now, and she says that her marriage and sex life are as good as ever. But she also says that as in any marriage, she and her husband have had ups and downs and times when things seemed to be falling apart. "When that happens," she says, "you work to put things back together again."

Her marriage is no different than millions of others, despite the fact that she's married to one of the most famous rock guitarists in the world— Saul Hudson, better known as Slash, solo artist and former lead guitarist of Guns N' Roses.

"Time, time, time is the recurrent theme in this marriage," says Perla. "You get caught up with children, your career, and running your household, and they get to be priorities over your husband, and you find that you've fallen into a rut that doesn't include sex. I always had good intentions of getting intimate with my husband, but we'd constantly get interrupted. My office would call, or the kids would need attention. I finally decided that if we wanted to have sex, we had to find a way to find the time."

She doesn't have a set "date night" in her calendar. Every so often, though, she takes a step back and realizes she hasn't had sex in a while, and then books a hotel room for herself and Slash. "The best part is that, unless it's an emergency, nobody is allowed to contact us while we're reconnecting and refueling."

If a hotel getaway is not a possibility, Perla has her own hideaway at home. She's turned her bedroom into a sexual sanctuary. The room, which includes a mirrored ceiling over the bed, is off limits to the kids. "I had a hand-crafted iron rod gate installed in the hallway leading up to the bedroom," she says. "I wanted a space where I could be completely uninhibited and where my little pumpkins couldn't somehow get by a locked door. The gate does the trick."

Perla also had a stripper pole installed in her bedroom and dances often for her husband. "I just couldn't lose the excess weight I put on after the children were born," she says, "and although my husband was still interested, I didn't feel sexy or sexual. I started pole dancing and not only did the weight fly off but I began to feel sexy again."

Perla has a couple of other secrets to keeping her sex life spicy. She wears sexy lingerie, and not always for her husband, but to turn herself on now that she feels comfortable wearing seductive things. Slash appreciates this as well. But her most effective secret is fantasizing—not about other men, but about what attracted her to Slash in the first place. "Then I go back in my mind to that time and place. It helps get me in the mood. Of course, the main thing that keeps us going after all this time," she says, "is that we're still in love."

WHY GOOD SEX IS GREAT FOR YOUR HEALTH

In my professional practice, I see many women who would be very happy never to have sex again. That is not to say they don't want relationships or to have romance in their lives. There's a difference between romance (which has more to do with emotional attachment) and sex. Do women want romance in their lives? Yes. Do they want intercourse? Not always.

It's entirely normal for sexual response to change dramatically over the course of a lifetime depending on hormone levels, lifestyle, health conditions, and environmental stress. Furthermore, the ultimate realization of the sexual response, the female orgasm, is a highly complicated emotional, mental, and physical event.

In fact, researchers have found that 33 to 50 percent of women experience orgasm infrequently and are dissatisfied with how often they reach orgasm. In addition, 10 to 15 percent of American women have *never* experienced an orgasm. During intercourse, only 35 percent of the female population climaxes. These statistics say a lot about the state of women's sexuality today.

I have spent my career studying the effects of metabolism and hormones on the emotional and spiritual dimensions of female sexuality. If you are less than satisfied with your sexual response, you will find various strategies in the following pages to start upgrading it. But maybe you're not concerned about your lack of libido. Maybe you're simply willing to accept it as part of being a busy working mother or just as a consequence of growing older. Don't fall into that trap! Don't give up on yourself and your own enjoyment and your own health—because what you may not know is that, for a variety of reasons, sexual activity is actually good for you. Let's take a look at some of the major reasons why you stand to benefit from regular, safe sex.

Much persuasive research shows that sexual activity enhances female as well as male health. You should have sex as often as possible, because an active sex life is a form of health insurance. This holds true even if you're having sex on your own. Why? Because masturbating to orgasm has been documented as providing various health benefits. While some people want more sex than others, only *you* can define what the right frequency is for you and your relationship (but *zero* shouldn't be one of your options). Frequency is subjective, and it's important to point out that many health-care professionals define "sexless" marriage as less than ten incidents of sexual intercourse in the past twelve months. This level of frequency may, however, feel right for you and your partner. Any less, however, should be looked into. In the final analysis, it's about quality and your contentment. Here is a short list of the health and well-being benefits of having sex:

❖ **Sex burns calories.** Making love is like any other exercise in that the longer your heart rate is maintained at a higher than normal "resting" rate, the more calories you will burn. Sexual activity, including masturbation, helps burn calories and fat, according to studies cited in Planned Parenthood's 2003 publication, "The Health Benefits of Sexual Expression." Enjoying safe sexual intercourse three times a week or more can burn anywhere from 200 to 600 calories. This in turn will help keep the weight off while promoting improved blood circulation, oxygen flow, and the release of the body's own natural pain-killing hormones. While intensity of sexual exertion differs from one individual to the next, even slow, leisurely sex is enough activity to raise your heart above its normal rate because of the hormones that are released during the excitation. If maintained throughout the year, the caloric expenditure involved in having intercourse three times a week may be equivalent to jogging 75 miles. And making love is so much more fun than jogging, right?

❖ **Sex increases oxygenation.** Researchers have known for decades that sex can not only be as beneficial as other forms of exercise in raising the heart rate, it can also promote enhanced blood flow and respiration. The increase in the rate at which blood and air circulate corresponds to a greater supply of oxygen throughout the body, which is vital for optimal organ and tissue health. More oxygen in the body means that we are less susceptible to opportunistic bacteria, viral, and parasitic infections, colds and flus, and even cancer. An added benefit is that sexual activity causes your blood vessels to dilate, and you send lots of blood closer to the surface of your skin. At the same time, your body pumps a lot of oxygen into your red blood cells. Many women, and some men, experience what is called a "sex flush" just before and during orgasm. And as it turns out, more blood and oxygen in skin is attractive to others. A recent study by researchers from the University of St. Andrews in Scotland found that men selected photos of women featuring a slightly rosier glow as being more attractive. So you might want to consider a little solo satisfaction just before you head out for that big date. Who needs makeup when you can let your natural rosy glow shine through!

❖ **Sex promotes cardiovascular health.** Regular sexual release can help protect your heart, according to a study published in the medical journal *Psychosomatic Medicine*. Women who cannot experience orgasm are more likely to develop heart disease and experience heart attacks than orgasmic women. If more women were making love more often, this could make a potentially life-saving and certainly life-enhancing difference in the epidemic of female heart disease plaguing the United States.

❖ **Sex boosts immunity.** College students in Wilkes-Barre, PA, took part in a study in which they reported the frequency of sex they had. Those students who reported sexual activity once or twice a week had 30 percent higher levels of an antibody called immunoglobulin A, or IgA, which can protect you from getting colds and other infections.

❖ **Sex relieves stress and depression.** Sexual activity relaxes the nervous, respiratory, and circulatory systems, according to a study conducted by Roy J. Levin of the University of Sheffield in Sheffield, England. Levin reports that hormones in semen contain substances that have been found to relax a woman, which is one reason we often feel in a better mood after a man ejaculates inside the vagina. Another study found that participants who had had intercourse were better able to handle stress in many situations (including public speaking and doing verbal arithmetic) than those who had not had intercourse. And a 2002 American study conducted by psychologist Gordon Gallup found that women whose male partners did not use condoms suffered less depression than those whose partners did wear condoms. I do not, obviously, advocate unsafe sex to cure depression; however, if you are in a long-term monogamous relationship and both of you have been tested for sexually transmitted diseases, then you might want to experiment to see if not using a condom makes a difference. The theory is that prostaglandin, a hormone found in semen, gets absorbed in the female genital tract, thus modulating female hormones. And we know that sex releases brain endorphins, which automatically lifts your mood and helps relieve stress.

❖ **Sex optimizes fertility and helps maintain vaginal youth.** It has also been found that regular deposits of seminal fluid in the vagina make a woman more likely to ovulate on a regular basis, thus optimizing her fertility. In postmenopausal women, semen appears to assist in counteracting vaginal atrophy, a condition characterized by the drying and shrinking of the vaginal lining, which can result in vaginal discomfort and pain during intercourse.

❖ **Sex relieves menstrual cramps.** As you may already know from personal experience, sexual release can help relieve menstrual cramps. This has been documented in various studies and was reported in the 2003 Planned Parenthood report. Planned Parenthood also reported that orgasm causes a surge in the calming hormone oxytocin (a natural chemical in the body that surges before and during climax) and feel-good hormones, such as endorphins, that may act as sedation. They cite a study which found that 32 percent of 1,866 U.S. women who reported masturbating in the previous three months did so to help them go to sleep. Another study reported that 9 percent of about 1,900 U.S. women who reported masturbating in the previous three months cited relief of menstrual cramps as a motivation.

❖ **Sexual activity may prevent endometriosis.** One breakthrough study conducted at the Yale School of Medicine suggests that sexual activity might prevent endometriosis, a painful condition that affects an estimated ten million American women and often results in infertility. The endometrium is the uterine lining and normally grows only in the uterus, exiting the body each month during menstruation. In endometriosis, endometrial tissue grows in the fallopian tubes, ovaries, and other pelvic parts, and in rare cases, outside of the pelvis. Endometriosis typically afflicts women who are childless or those who have children late in life. Fascinating new research also indicates that women with shorter menstrual cycles and longer periods are also at a higher risk. According to the Yale study, women who had sexual intercourse during menstruation were *one and a half times less likely* to develop endometriosis than women who never made love during their periods. Having sex during your period may actually positively impact your fertility by reducing the likelihood of developing endometriosis. The researchers also found that *orgasm during menstruation lowered the risk of developing endometriosis.* This is key information since the backup of menstrual fluid in the pelvic cavity is currently believed to play a pivotal role in the development of endometriosis. It's possible that contractions of the uterus during lovemaking, and specifically orgasm, may help push menstrual material out of the uterus.

Those Fabulous Follow-Me Pheromones

Many people say that it's chemistry that attracts two people to each other. In Africa, they say that some animals have "follow-me pheromones" (chemical signals that trigger a natural response in another member of the same species) that are emitted during mating season. The jury is actually still out as to whether or not humans emit pheromones, although it can sometimes seem the only explanation for how and why certain people choose their sexual and marital partners. In Western society, women often go after potential mates who have money and power. It is the same in nature, as females flock after the most powerful males. If you're looking for the secret to sexual attraction, it just might be mind over matter: believe in your follow-me pheromones and you might be pleasantly surprised!

SEX AND YOUR TRICKY HORMONES

Secreted in the brain and throughout the entire body are hormones called endorphins, similar in chemical structure to morphine. Endorphins are your body's built-in wonder drug. However, unlike morphine (and antidepressants), endorphins provide free, health-enhancing benefits without negative side effects.

Endorphins are released during orgasm and can provide varying degrees of pain relief. Oxytocin likely plays a role as well. According to a study conducted by sexologist Beverly Whipple, professor emeritus at Rutgers University, when women masturbated to orgasm "the pain tolerance threshold and pain detection threshold increased significantly by 74.6 percent and 106.7 percent respectively," as measured by a sensory device designed to produce a report of pressure vs. pleasure. With these encouraging results in mind, try pleasuring yourself sexually the next time you have a headache, instead of turning off. You very well may end up feeling fantastic and pain free.

Endorphins block pain signals from reaching the nervous system and thus are critical to maintaining optimum health. These substances produce physical feelings of well-being that translate into positive emotional and mental states. Consciously cultivating endorphin release (by masturbating or by having someone else stimulate your favorite spots—a soft kiss on the neck or behind the ear, for instance) gives you the power to literally turn yourself on whenever you want. In addition to curbing stress and anxiety and enhancing your body's immunity and disease-fighting capability, liberating your endorphins can help heighten sexual energy and libido.

These feel-good hormones can give you an overall energy boost as well as a sense of well-being that can last for several hours after the deed is done.

Unfortunately, we can't always rely on endorphins alone to regain that lovin' feeling. When men have a sexual "problem," it's pretty obvious. They can't get it up. Or they can't keep it up. Or they can get it partway up, but not as up as they'd like it to be. But women's sexual arousal is a much more complex—and in many ways more subtle—subject. Very little is known about how a woman's libido actually functions. There are many theories involving some or all of the following: hormones, brain chemicals such as serotonin and endorphins, external stimuli, and the competencies of sexual partners. There is no agreement, even among professionals in the field of human sexuality, as to what is "normal" for women to experience in terms of sexual desire or the lack thereof.

Luckily, things are beginning to change as women are more and more willing to acknowledge that their decreased libido has become an issue in their relationships. In years past, women were reluctant, mostly due to societal taboos, to talk about sexual issues. My mother certainly didn't (at least not to me). You just performed your "wifely duties" and didn't talk about your own satisfaction. In some ways, women have Viagra to thank for getting the conversation started on this issue. When erectile dysfunction came out of the closet, so to speak, women began to talk about their problems as well. In fact, I have many patients who come to me because they're looking for ways to keep up with their Viagra-popping significant others who suddenly want much more sex than they have in years. Right now, there is no equivalent drug for women. Some patients have experimented by trying their husband's Viagra but found it did not work. I would certainly not recommend that you try this, but there are definitely ways that women of all ages can address hormonal issues that may be slowing down or stopping their sexual responses.

The 411 on Sex Hormones

As we talked about earlier in the book, problems can develop when our hormones are out of balance. When our sex hormones are out of balance, they can cause sexual problems. While it is true that many hormonal changes are basically a result of the aging process, I see women of all ages with complaints of hormonal imbalances in my practice. If your sex hormones are imbalanced, you are most likely going to be tired all the time, you're going to be irritable and unhappy, and you're going to gain weight (which will make you even more tired, irritable, and unhappy).

The three main sex hormones are:

❖ **Estrogen:** A female sex hormone produced by the ovaries, the adrenal gland, and (in small quantities) by body fat. Estrogen helps to retain calcium in bones, regulates the balance of HDL and LDL cholesterol in the bloodstream, and aids the maintenance of blood-sugar levels, memory functions, and emotional balance, just to mention a few.

❖ **Progesterone:** A female sex hormone produced in largest amounts during and after ovulation that prepares the uterus for the implantation of a fertilized egg. It also helps reduce body fat, aids in relaxation and reduction of anxiety, and promotes hair growth.

❖ **Testosterone:** The principal male sex hormone, testosterone is also produced in smaller amounts in women's bodies mostly by the ovaries and adrenal glands. It plays an important role in the health and well-being. Testosterone affects libido, mood, energy, and body fat and helps to protect against osteoporosis.

When estrogen, progesterone, and testosterone are all doing their jobs, they work well together. They are regulated by a complicated feedback system that involves the hypothalamus, the pituitary gland, the ovaries, and the adrenal gland. Stress, nutrition, and exercise all affect that feedback system, and therefore affect your hormonal balance (see Chapter 9 on testing to find out how you can determine if you have a hormone imbalance).

Probably the most misunderstood hormone is testosterone. Few of my female patients understand the decisive role that testosterone plays in their lives and loves. Testosterone is critically important, functioning as the key substance influencing sexual desire in women.

Recently, Dolores, a 70-year-old patient of mine, alerted me to the fact that she and her husband had started sleeping in separate bedrooms. He had gained 30 pounds and started snoring, keeping her awake at night. Many 70-year-olds I see prefer to sleep in separate bedrooms from their husbands as an antidote for sleepless nights due to their husbands' snoring or thrashing about in bed (women are notoriously lighter sleepers than their counterparts). This may sound like a solution to the problem of getting a good night's rest, but studies show that when couples start sleeping apart, the incidence of divorce rises. Dolores was not pleased with this option. She told me that she wasn't having much of a sex life, but at least she was getting the sleep she needed.

When I first started practicing medicine it was odd, to say the least, for an elderly woman to even utter the word *sex*. But now, many older women are willing to discuss their problems in the bedroom. Dolores was on estrogen, so vaginal dryness (a problem for many older women) was not an issue. Her problem wasn't that of libido, it was that she had trouble having an orgasm. She really enjoyed intercourse, but had difficulty in climaxing.

I placed Dolores on topical bioidentical testosterone cream. I added Wellbutrin (an antidepressant known to increase orgasms in woman). After a month, Dolores came to my office and told me that her sex life was better now than it had been in over 20 years. She couldn't believe that she was back to her old sexy self. Her husband sent me flowers. Eventually, she convinced her husband to lose weight, he stopped snoring, and they moved back into the bedroom together.

Studies have shown that testosterone can be considered one of the most powerful natural antidepressants on the market. A recent study found that 6,000 women who had been on Prozac for depression were able to get off the drug after using a testosterone patch. Testosterone supplementation is a fantastic option since it's been proven to boost libido by making a woman think, feel, and act sexier.

Women in their 20s to mid-30s generally have healthy testosterone levels powering their libidos. Yet stress, poor diet, and other factors can diminish testosterone levels as women age, particularly as natural hormonal changes occur in their late 30s.

Most women over the age of 35 have little or no free testosterone, the hormone that is critically involved in fostering sexual arousal and well-being. This can account for the sexual energy crisis experienced by so many women in their mid- to late 30s. Common symptoms that often indicate low testosterone in women include general low energy, depression, weight gain, and feeling tired all the time and/or easily overwhelmed. Other possible indicators are brain fog, difficulty concentrating, feeling too stressed or too time-crunched to have sex, premenstrual syndrome problems (bloating, headaches, fatigue, moodiness, skin changes, heart palpitations, and shortness of breath) and difficult perimenopause or postmenopausal symptoms (weight gain—especially in the midabdominal section—mood changes, and insomnia). Remember, it's normal to have an abnormal level of testosterone as you age.

Total Testosterone vs. Free Testosterone

Do you have any symptoms of low testosterone levels mentioned above? If you do, you may want to go to your doctor and get tested for testosterone. Most likely your results will show your total testosterone levels. Even women in their 70s often have "normal" total testosterone levels. The level you're really looking for is of free testosterone. In women, only about 1 to 3 percent of total testosterone is made up of free testosterone; the rest is attached to proteins in the blood. It is only the free or nonprotein-bound testosterone, which is the hormonally active form, able to interact with cellular hormone receptors.

Prior to prescribing a testosterone regimen, I always administer tests to ensure my patient is a good candidate for the treatment and that there are no risk factors (women who are of child-bearing age should not take testosterone. See page 151 for supplements appropriate for women who are still considering having children). I then monitor them closely for some time after initiating treatment.

Not only may testosterone supplementation increase libido and facilitate climax, testosterone also helps convert fat into muscle, a fact that most women can heartily appreciate. Studies have shown that transdermal (applied directly to the skin) testosterone applied as a cream can reduce the need for higher levels of estrogen replacement in women who have night sweats and hot flashes.

Testosterone can be given as a cream (it is one of the most commonly prescribed substances in my practice), although some women prefer to choose other delivery systems such as testosterone tablets, injections, implantable pellets, sublingual (under the tongue) drops, and lozenges, to name a few. Many patients tell me that testosterone gives them more energy for work, family, and exercise, and it often helps them lose weight. In addition to making women generally more productive, the increase in physical and sexual energy, coupled with weight loss, helps raise self-esteem, and improves overall quality of life.

Of course, as with anything else, testosterone supplementation has possible side effects. For less than 2 percent of people taking it, testosterone can produce acne, oily skin, excess body hair, or other masculinizing effects. These can usually be counteracted by changing the dose of the testosterone. No studies as of this writing have shown that it is associated with breast cancer or with stroke.

There is no one-size-fits-all solution for loss of libido. Women who are willing to try testosterone therapy may have to go through a trial-and-error period with their health-care professional to find the dose and delivery system that is best for them.

From Dr. Eva's Files

Linda is an attractive 49-year-old woman who went through menopause three years ago. She has been divorced for more than 20 years. When she came to see me with symptoms of lingering lethargy and a general feeling of being off her game, I asked about her love life.

"Love life?" she said. "I haven't had sex in 20 years." After testing found that her testosterone levels were quite low, I prescribed a low dose for her to start on. A few weeks later, I got an early morning

phone call from Linda. She was in Russia, she'd met a man, and they had sex. She also had a rip-roaring headache. I assured her that it was due to the unfamiliar surge of energy and hormones going on in her body, and told her to relax and enjoy the experience. When she returned to see me after her trip, I asked if she wanted to be taken off the testosterone. "Hell, no," she said. "I'm having too much fun. I can always take an aspirin for the headache."

Hormones and the Pill

When female patients come to me for help with low or nonexistent libido, the first question I ask them is whether they are on the birth-control pill, and if so, which one. That's because very few women today are aware of how birth-control pills may be sapping their energy and dampening their sex lives.

Most birth-control pills today contain 21 to 24 active pills and 4 to 7 placebo pills. The active pills are made up of a combination of estrogen and progestin (there is a "minipill" that contains only progesterone, which is designed for women who are breastfeeding or who have conditions that prevent them from taking estrogen). There are basically three types of combination birth-control pills available by prescription today:

- ❖ Monophasic: these pills (including brand names such as Brevicon, Loestrin, and Norinyl) contain equal amounts of estrogen and progestin in each pill.

- ❖ Biphasic: these pills (including brand names such as Kariva, Mircette, and Ortho-Novum 10/11) contain two different levels of estrogen and progestin.

- ❖ Triphasic: these pills (including brand names such as Ortho-Novum 7/7/7, Tri-Levlen, and Tri-Norinyl) contain three different concentrations of estrogen and progestin that vary throughout the menstrual cycle.

Who Should You See?

If you are dealing with loss of libido, I generally recommend that you see an endocrinologist rather than depend on your general practitioner or gynecologist. A general practitioner or primary-care physician doesn't usually offer the necessary in-depth laboratory testing nor will he or she know how to properly interpret the results. Even gynecologists, who may be better informed about hormones, don't usually have the same level of knowledge about them as an endocrinologist. Even when choosing an endocrinologist, it's important to do your homework, as there are several subspecialties in the field.

Some endocrinologists deal only with thyroid issues (check out www .thyroid-info.com for a list of thyroid specialists in your state and patients' comments about these doctors), others only deal with diabetes or pituitary tumors. If you're looking for help with special issues, call the doctor's office and ask the receptionist what portion of the practice is devoted to issues such as yours. Also, speak to your friends and ask if they have any recommendations since all these issues are prevalent in our society and someone else you know is sure to have investigated the options. Always do your own research as well (not just online). Ask what the doctor's true training is in (you want to be sure the doctor isn't an anesthesiologist who has decided to practice hormone-replacement therapy on his own, for instance). Although some doctors may be certified to practice antiaging medicine through organizations such as the American Board of Holistic Medicine and a few may be brilliant at what they do, there is no antiaging board-certified specialty recognized by the American Medical Association or the American Board of Medical Specialties.

A relatively new addition to the birth-control-pill family is the extended-cycle pill, with brand names including Seasonale and Seasonique. They, too, are combination pills containing both estrogen and progestin. However, you take these pills for extended periods of time, which means you get your period once every three or four months.

Although the pill itself contains no testosterone, persuasive research has shown that women who use oral contraceptive pills may develop long-term sexual health problems because their bodies are filled with low amounts of "unbound," or free, testosterone, which is bad news for women as it can potentially lead to continuing negative sexual, metabolic, and mental health consequences, including a flat libido.

Put another way, the birth-control pill increases the number of sex hormone binding globulins (SHBG) so that they attach to testosterone more readily, leaving less testosterone to freely circulate through the body—making us less horny.

When the birth-control pill first became available in the early 60s, it created the sexual revolution. We could now have sex without worrying about getting pregnant. We could have sex whenever we wanted. What we weren't prepared for was that now that we could have unbridled sex, we didn't really want to! Nobody was talking about the fact that the chronic elevation of SHBG levels from using the pill may in fact cause decreased desire, decreased arousal, decreased lubrication, and increased sexual pain. Even today, it's rarely talked about. When you go to see your gynecologist to get on the pill, you almost never hear the doctor say, "By the way, taking this pill may cause loss of libido." If it's discussed at all, it's usually after the fact. A typical scenario goes like this:

Patient: "I stopped taking the birth-control pill"
Doctor: "Why?"
Patient: "My boyfriend broke up with me. He thought I didn't love him anymore because I lost interest in him. It happened soon after I started taking the pill. Do you think it may be related?"
Doctor: "Why yes, it is certainly a possibility."
Patient: "Well, I sure wish you had told me that in the first place! He was the love of my life. Now all I do is feel sorry for myself and eat junk food all day. I lost my job because I was so depressed over him, and developed horrible acne over that stress so now no one wants to date me."

Don't get me wrong. I am a firm believer in the pill as it allows a woman to have spontaneous sex with her partner without the risk of unplanned pregnancy. However, as a doctor, I urge my patients to discuss the various types of birth-control pills on the market today, and which one might be best for them. Choosing the appropriate pill and closely monitoring a woman's reaction is critical in maintaining peak emotional, sexual, and physical health. Side effects can include weight gain, emotional irritability, hair loss, acne, gastric reflux, constipation, and decreased sex drive. If you are adversely affected by a low libido then at least you'll know it's because of the pill and not necessarily because of the relationship itself.

One 1996 study out of San Francisco State University, however, found that the type of pill you take can make a difference. Researchers found that those women on triphasic pills had higher sex drives, more sexual fantasies, and were generally more aroused during sex than those on other forms of birth control. Researchers were not sure exactly why triphasic pills had this effect; it could possibly be due to the fact that triphasic pills contain a slightly lower amount of progestin than other combination pills. There are now many options for women, and you may have to try more than one before you find what's right for you.

That being said, I usually recommend a monophasic pill for several reasons: it provides the same amount of hormones throughout the cycle, which means there are fewer mood swings; women bleed for a maximum of four days a month, which is a lifestyle benefit; and it causes less weight gain than other types of pills. Perhaps most important for our purposes, monophasic birth control decreases libido less than biphasic or triphasic pills. Monophasic pills don't affect sex hormone binding globulin (SHBG) as much as the others do, which means it has less binding potential with testosterone—in other words, one stays hornier when taking monophasic birth control.

Is My Antacid Affecting My Sex Drive?

Birth-control pills are not the only medications that can cause loss of libido. Many prescription medications can have the same effect, including hypertension medications, beta blockers, antiseizure medications, Prozac, and Paxil. Even over-the-counter medications such as antacids (including Zantac, Tums, Mylanta) and antihistamines (including Zyrtec and Benadryl) can cause you to say, "Sorry, hon, not tonight." Antacids neutralize the acid production in your digestive system; acid is actually necessary for the absorption of certain nutrients needed to produce hormones. Antihistamines can make you tired, and they can blunt the receptors that usually work to stimulate orgasm. So if you suddenly find yourself uninterested and can't figure out why, check with your doctor. It just might be a new medication that's giving you a headache—literally or figuratively.

READY . . . SET . . . RECHARGE!

Once you've checked out your hormones and perhaps received the treatment you need, your next step is to keep and maintain the intimacy, playfulness, and romance you had when you and your partner first got together. The nature of your relationship changes over the years, and familiarity and complacency may creep into your lives in place of the bloom of first love. That's only to be expected and even acknowledged. But that doesn't mean you just say, "Oh, well," and give up. There are plenty of things you can do to keep your love life rewarding and energetic. Here are just a few.

TALK ABOUT IT

Most women who are not having satisfactory sex lives feel isolated in their circumstances. They feel as if everyone else is having great sex, and they're the only ones who aren't. The truth is that millions of women are in the same situation. It may be a good idea to talk to your friends and ask them how they feel about their sex lives. Do it with humor—and maybe a glass or two of wine— and you may be surprised to find out that they feel the same way you do. Or if they feel differently, they may be able to give you some ideas about how they're spicing up their love lives.

If you're not comfortable with that, find a health professional or therapist to talk to. A lot of people are nervous when they go to see a doctor. It's understandable—nobody likes feeling ill or wondering if they have a serious disease that will turn their lives upside down. Let me give you an example. Iris had been my patient for several years, and I knew that, other than some relatively minor hormone balance issues, she was in good shape. So I was very concerned when she came in for a routine follow-up visit appearing pale, shaky, and unable to look me in the eye. It took some gentle persuasion, but I finally got her to tell me what was wrong. As it turned out, Iris and her husband of ten years were having problems in bed. More and more frequently, she was just too tired and he couldn't get an erection. But the worst part was that Iris was sure it was because she wasn't desirable enough to keep him interested, or even worse, that he was seeing another woman. She felt that she couldn't talk to her friends because they all seemed so secure in their relationships (Well, there was her one friend who was getting a divorce but surely it couldn't have anything to do with sexual issues. Her friend was beautiful, after all.) So, embarrassed as she was, Iris came to see me so I could tell her what was wrong.

I assured her there was nothing abnormal about her situation, that we would test her hormone levels to make sure nothing had gone haywire in her system (and if it had, we would fix it), and most of all, I commended her for talking to me about it. There's no reason for Iris, or anyone else, to suffer in silence about a problem that has such an impact on quality of life. Long story short, she finally had the good sense to discuss the situation with her husband, who was relieved that she did. It turned out that the problem was actually a hormone imbalance with her husband (but that's a story for the next book), and he was grateful that she persuaded him to go to the doctor and get it checked out. Their marriage is now stronger and sexier than ever. You see, it's not always the woman who has the problem. By encouraging open conversation regarding matters of the bedroom, most problems can be solved.

Don't be embarrassed to speak to your doctor or health practitioner about your concerns. Keep in mind that your doctor has probably had this conversation with dozens if not hundreds or even thousands of other patients. This is confidential information; it's not gossip that gets spread around or office talk after you have left an appointment. You already have an "intimate" relationship with your doctor—he or she has probably seen you naked, and if that doctor has done a pap smear or a rectal exam, how much more intimate can you get? A good doctor will make you feel comfortable enough to discuss anything. And if that doctor doesn't feel he can help, he can at least refer you to an appropriate specialist. You don't have to be embarrassed or feel guilty. This is a very common situation.

And what you may not realize is that your partner is probably feeling just the same way. Talk about it. Share your concerns. Perhaps together you can come up with ways to improve the situation—such as the jump-start tips at the end of this chapter.

Give a Massage

You don't have to be a professional masseuse to make someone else feel good. A simple back or shoulder rub can be exceedingly sensual. If your partner enjoys massage, it can be a great way to start a romantic evening. This is also a good opportunity to find out (or to rediscover) just how your partner likes to be touched. Some people enjoy a light touch, while others appreciate a deeper rubdown. It's usually easiest to start with your partner lying face down on the bed while you start massaging the neck and shoulders where most people store a lot of tension. If you find a spot where your partner likes to be rubbed, chances are he or she will like to be kissed there as well. Experiment with massage oils, many of which are edible. And try playing some calming music in the background. One more option is to sit behind your lover in the bathtub and give your massage there. The warm water can add a super-sexy feeling. Of course, your partner can return the favor immediately, or promise that tomorrow night will be your turn.

Try Acupuncture

Within acupuncture, a low libido is seen as an imbalance of chi within the organ systems, specifically the kidney and heart systems. According to the Mayo Clinic, about 40 percent of women will complain of a loss of sexual desire at some point in their lives. Many of the libido problems in women are a result of hormonal imbalances, and acupuncture has been proven to be effective in the treatment of these conditions. Acupuncture has been shown to help a variety of sexual problems for both men and women. It has also been used to help alleviate hot flashes and other symptoms of menopause.

I usually recommend acupuncture to women who don't have an obvious hormone imbalance or for whom hormone therapy is inappropriate. Typically, they go twice a week for three or four weeks, and then every other week for as long as it is helping them.

Watch an X-rated Movie

Men seem to love these things. I mean really love them. So you might want to see if it does anything for you. If you hate it, then don't use this as a romantic aid. Many women believe that women don't watch porn. But in the first three months of 2007, according to Nielsen/NetRatings, approximately one in three visitors to adult entertainment Web sites was female; during the same period nearly 13 million American women were checking out porn online at least once a month. And, in a 2006 study at McGill University, researchers monitored temperature changes of the genitals to show sexual arousal. They found that when they were shown clips of X-rated films, men and women alike began displaying arousal within 30 seconds. Men reached maximum arousal in about 11 minutes, women in about 12. If you've never seen a pornographic movie before, you might want to watch one by yourself. It doesn't make you a deviant, and it can be a once-in-a-while "guilty pleasure" for you and your partner if you both get pleasure from it. Many women tell me they have never gotten through a whole movie with their mate—the movie barely gets started when they start to get bare.

21st Century Kama Sutra

The *Kama Sutra* is an ancient sex manual written and rewritten over the course of centuries. It has been a literary classic for 1,700 years and is based on the premise that everyone can benefit from helpful and enlightening notes on "the right way to live." It's time to update the *Kama Sutra*'s advice using evidence-based medical research. We begin with the power of scent. The power of scent and its ability to effect psychological and sexual changes is one of the *Kama Sutra*'s recurring themes and has been qualified by modern science. Tapping into the power of scent to enhance attraction and lovemaking can be easily, quickly, and inexpensively accomplished by placing fresh cut flowers around the bedroom, sprinkling fragrant flower petals on pillows and sheets, or by using essential oils in bath water or in diffusers placed in the bedroom.

Interestingly, certain fragrant scents can also create positive impressions of us in the minds of others. According to studies conducted by Alan R. Hirsch at the Smell & Taste Treatment and Research Center in Chicago, women who wore lemony or other citrus-scented fragrances tended to be perceived by men as being younger than their actual age by five to seven years while spicy-floral scents were found to make others perceive women as weighing as much as twelve pounds less than their actual weight. Dr. Hirsch's team of researchers also found that jasmine fosters receptivity in men so you may try applying jasmine essential oil before going on a date. Lavender and pumpkin pie spice were found to be the most sexually arousing scents to men and enhanced penile blood flow accordingly. In the *Kama Sutra* and other ancient literature, cinnamon is used as a perfume to lure men into romantic embrace.

Of course, the *Kama Sutra* contains a good deal more than the power of scent. It also details a variety of sexual positions designed to bring pleasure to both parties. It is a beautiful book that can function as a guide as well as an ice breaker. If you're shy, it can be a great way to open up lines of communication.

If you're looking for more modern sex guides, there are a wide variety on the market today that can be both fun and educational, such as:

❖ *The Enlightened Sex Manual: Sexual Skills for the Superior Lover* by David Deida

❖ *The Sex Bible: The Complete Guide to Sexual Love* by Susan Crain Bakos

❖ *Discovering Your Couple Sexual Style: Sharing Desire, Pleasure, and Satisfaction* by Barry W. McCarthy and Emily McCarthy

And don't forget about erotic magazines or novels. It can be very stimulating to take turns reading to each other, or reading by yourself. What you read depends on your personal level of comfort—it's good to push the envelope a little bit, but not so much that it ends up being distasteful and turning you off instead of turning you on.

A Room with a Viewpoint

If you want your bedroom to be conducive to recharging your love life, try a little feng shui. Feng shui ("fung shway") is the art of creating a home environment that supports the life you wish to live. A key element of feng shui is creating a smooth flow of chi (positive energy) throughout your home—including your bedroom. Here are a few feng shui tips for creating sexual energy in the bedroom:

❖ Place romantic images in two key places in the bedroom: the wall opposite the foot of the bed (so you can see it when lying in bed), and whatever area of the room you first see when you enter. It can be a romantic painting, fresh or silk flowers, or erotic sculpture.

❖ Don't exercise in the bedroom or you will bring the energy of hard work and exertion into your romance space.

❖ Decorate with warm colors, beiges, reds, apricots, and yellows. Red, the color of love and passion, is best for sexual energy. Yellow is also another very good color for the bedroom because it symbolizes communication. Include soft furnishings and a comfortable bed in the room.

❖ Remove all clutter so positive energy can flow throughout the room. Clutter blocks the flow of chi.

❖ Display photos of you and your partner doing things together. Avoid having too many photos of friends or family members. The bedroom is a place for you to share with your loved one. Family pictures belong in the family room.

Aphrodisiac, Anyone?

Another beautifully woven theme running through the *Kama Sutra* is the sensual power of food and drink to enhance receptivity, forge intimacy, and heighten romance. Follow the wisdom of the *Kama Sutra* and share cinnamon-spiced foods such as butternut squash soup, cinnamon glazed carrots, apple pie, and cinnamon cookies. Enjoy licorice candies and flavor your drinking water with cucumber slices. More contemporary aphrodisiacs for consumption include mineral water flavored with pomegranate juice, champagne, organic red wine, and energizing fruits such as goji berries, raspberries, and crisp Asian pears. Dark chocolate, when enjoyed in moderation, confers health-enhancing benefits that make it a particularly enjoyable libido lifter. According to a study published in the *Journal of the American College of Nutrition,* small daily doses of flavonoid-rich dark chocolate consumed over a two-week period improved blood vessels' ability to expand, thus promoting greater blood flow throughout the brain and body and forging a healthier heart.

Replace Your After-Dinner Drink

Many people like to have a drink or two with dinner to get them in a romantic mood. That's great, but here's what really happens. You have a glass of wine at 7:00 or 8:00, then two or three hours later when you're ready to go to bed, you're too tired and all you want to do is go to sleep. Reserve that wine until after the kids are asleep, you've already finished discussing the day's events and the state of your finances, and you're actually ready for a little romance.

Sex from the Right Side of the Brain

You may be intrigued to know that one side of your brain literally feels happier than the other. The brain's left side is more optimistic and cheerful while the right tends to feel more negative, pessimistic, anxious, and sad.

As Dr. Daniel G. Amen notes in his book *Sex on the Brain,* women wanting to make a sexy and positive impression should remember to always stand to the right side of the object of their affection. When you stand to someone's right side, their experience of you is processed in the left and happier, more optimistic side of the brain.

It's fun to experiment with various romantic applications of this right-side advantage. For example, when taking a seat at a dinner party, sit to the right of the person you are most interested in. Sitting there may make them respond more warmly to your conversation and appearance. Likewise, when you are getting ready to retire for the night, lie down on your partner's right side. In amorous situations, stroking someone's right hand will excite them more than if their left hand is caressed and the same is true for kissing on the right side.

Trying these right-side suggestions and paying attention to how your lover reacts can give you a deeper experience of touch and sexual response. Ask your lover to touch you on your right side and see how it feels as compared to being touched on the other side. Brain imaging research at the University of Kuopio in Finland and elsewhere has documented that orgasmic experience appears to be primarily processed in the right hemisphere of the brain. The good news for women is that they tend to have greater access than men to the right side of the brain.

A Bold Move: G-Spot Amplification

Imagine being able to enhance the quality of your orgasms simply by having a quick and nearly painless injection in a doctor's office. The G-spot amplification shot allows you to do this. Designed strictly for sexual enhancement, this procedure has helped thousands of women dramatically improve their sexual satisfaction. This is a controversial procedure and is not approved by the FDA, mainly because there is no consensus as to where the G-spot is, or even if it really exists. I have included it here just to let you know that there are indeed a wide variety of options for women who are interested in improving their sex lives.

According to some experts, the G-spot is located in the anterior vaginal wall, about 2 or 3 centimeters in front of the cervix, near the bladder neck. This area's texture feels different from the rest of the vaginal interior as it softly ribbed, like corduroy material. However, according to Dr. Dolores Kent, a Los Angeles–based pioneer in specialized vaginal procedures, the G-spot is not an anatomical landmark. It's more of a zone than a spot. Many women (and their partners) go through life never knowing where their G-spot is, which is unfortunate because caressing and pressing lightly on this spot can lead to intense sexual arousal and orgasms.

The procedure starts with the physician locating the G-spot using a specially designed speculum to take measurements. Next, a local anesthetic is injected into the area where the G-spot has been located. Once the anesthetic has taken effect a synthetically engineered human collagen is injected into the G-spot, creating a marble-sized nub that pushes up against the spot. Dr. Kent states, "Four hours later, the woman is good to go. She can make love that night, and the benefits of the procedure last for about three months." This is not for women who don't have orgasms at all, but for women who want to enhance the sensations they already have. Many of her patients are women in their 30s who describe their sexual satisfaction level as a 6 before the procedure, and as a 10 after it is done.

The cost of the shot varies from physician to physician, averaging about $1,600.00. While Viagra, penile injections, and prosthesis for men are covered by most health-insurance plans to enhance male sexual fulfillment, G-spot amplification is still considered elective cosmetic surgery and therefore not yet covered by health plans. However, as long as you are practicing safe sex with your partner, the cost may be justified, as great sex is so beneficial for your physical and mental health.

Try Yoga

Certain forms of yoga believe that sexual experience is a means to enlightenment. Tantric yoga maintains that there is an enormous energy locked into sexuality, which, if released from the lower end of the spine, can flow up the spinal column to bring divine illumination to the brain. Sexual energy is considered the most concentrated form of biochemical energy in the human body. Here is an example of one exercise that is designed specifically to raise sexual energy:

1. Kneel on the floor, then sit back on your heels with your back straight.

2. Stretch your arms straight up so that your upper arms are hugging your ears. Clasp your hands together and interlace your fingers, except for the index finger of each hand. The index fingers are pointed straight up and pressed together.

3. Speak the word *sat* as you pull your naval up and in toward your spine. Also contract your rectum and sex organ. Let out your breath and relax your muscles as you say the word *nam*. Continue this repetition for at least three minutes, then inhale and squeeze the muscles tightly from the buttocks all the way up the back, past the shoulders. When you are done, lie on your back and rest for several minutes.

Try Meditation

A study conducted by psychologist Lori Brotto of the British Columbia Center for Sexual Medicine in Vancouver focused on the practice of mindfulness, a Buddhist technique of meditation in which you reach a mental state characterized by calm awareness of whatever you happen to be experiencing at the time. For example, many women who complain of loss of libido say that they are detached from their physical feelings during sex, distracted by the many tasks they have to accomplish the next day, worries about their children, or concerns about their careers. Brotto encourages them instead to notice and focus on physical sensations and to repeat phrases such as "My body is alive and sexual" whether they believe it or not. Many of the women reported stronger libidos and improved relationships.

"HOT PLANTS" AND SUPPLEMENTS FOR SEXUAL VIBRANCY

While synthetic and bioidentical hormones can work wonders for some women, there are also some naturally derived remedies that can boost libido and provide superb results. If you are not comfortable taking estrogen-replacement therapy or have special concerns or contraindications that make you want to bypass supplemental hormones, it's good to know there are options. It is very important to keep in mind that each woman's body chemistry is unique and may react differently to certain herbs. *Always* discuss with your physician before starting any herb or supplementation regimen.

With these variables in mind, let's take a look at some herbs that may help you ramp up sexual vitality:

❖ **Maca:** A hardy plant root that comes from the Andes Mountains. It holds great potential for helping to reduce debilitating symptoms of menstruation, perimenopause, menopause, and postmenopause. Patients taking maca report that it engenders a feeling of core strength and energy. It may be difficult to find maca in your local store, and there is a huge disparity in the quality of maca that is available. Be sure you read the labels and buy a reputable brand.

❖ **Tribulus:** It is traditionally used as a dietary supplement to increase energy, provide a healthier sex drive and better appetite, lower body fat levels, and improve athletic performance. It may increase testosterone levels in women but not enough to cause masculinizing effects. It can also be used to manage symptoms of menopause such as hot flashes, perspiration, insomnia, and low libido.

❖ **Ginseng:** Regarded throughout Asia as a supreme tonic for over 3000 years, ginseng has been used to help strengthen organs, glands, and energy systems. Today, people around the world take ginseng to tune up health and sexual well-being as well as build endurance for physical exercise, high altitudes, airplane travel, etc. Ginseng should be taken on a daily basis for at least several months because like all herbs, its effects are cumulative. *Please note that ginseng is not recommended for those with high blood pressure.*

❖ **Arginine:** Plays an important role in cell division, the healing of wounds, removing ammonia from the body, immune function, and the release of hormones. Arginine has also been used as a treatment for erectile dysfunction. It increases blood circulation throughout the body, including the sex organs, and has been shown to improve reproductive ability

❖ **DHEA:** DHEA is a hormone that is secreted throughout the body during sex. At orgasm, DHEA levels in the bloodstream increase to five times normal. Secreted by the adrenal cortex (the outer portion of the adrenal gland located on top of each kidney), this steroid is necessary for the production of testosterone in humans. High levels of DHEA have been associated with longevity, enhanced libido, increased muscle mass, and decreased depression. Studies have shown DHEA supplementation to improve subjective mood and decrease evening cortisol concentration, which is known to be elevated in depression.

❖ **5-HTP:** The metabolic precursor to the neurotransmitter serotonin. Tryptophan, an essential amino acid, is metabolized into 5-HTP by the body. 5-HTP is, in turn, converted into the serotonin, which regulates sleep, anxiety, depression, sexual behavior, pain sensation, and appetite. 5-HTP is manufactured from the seeds of the African plant *Griffonia simplicifolia*. Some antidepressant drugs, including selective serotonin reuptake inhibitors (SSRIs) such as Prozac, are said to work by increasing the amount of serotonin available to the brain. 5-HTP, therefore, may serve for some people as a natural alternative to some prescription SSRI-type drugs.

❖ **"Green" Juice Products:** The most common substances found in green juice products are blue-green algae, wheat grass, barley grass, oat grass, spirulina (a form of algae), chlorella (also a form of algae), and dulse (seaweed). Green juice products contain many physiologically fortifying nutrients and are rich in trace minerals, the catalysts that enable vitamins and enzymes to perform their various functions. They also may supply essential amino acids that cannot be manufactured by the body yet are vital to health and sexual functioning. Green juice products are among the few common nutritional sources of chlorophyll, which functions to activate the enzymes that produce vitamins E, A, and K. Chlorophyll has a structure that is almost identical to that of hemoglobin, a naturally occurring substance that carries oxygen throughout the body. More oxygen means more energy for your body to enjoy a healthy sex life.

All of the supplements listed here are available without prescription. They all have manufacturers' suggested dosages on the bottles. Never take more than the recommended dosage, and always check with your health-care professional before you start taking any of these as some may react with medications you are already taking or conditions you may have.

THE SEXUAL ENERGY
jump-start tips

I know how many of you are anxious and excited to get this part of your life back into the high-energy zone. Keep in mind that reviving your sexual desire is in some ways like starting an exercise program. Most of us don't really want to go to the gym, but once we get there we actually enjoy it. The more we go, the more we begin to look forward to the pleasure we're going to experience when we're done. These steps are meant to help you get your libido back on track. What that means is individual to your own personal expectations. If you haven't been having sex at all, and the jump start helps you have sex once a week, that's great. If you've been having sex regularly but want to ramp things up, use these steps to help you get out of your sexual rut. There's no magic formula or relationship rule that says you have to have sex (with a partner or by yourself) a certain number of times a week to be healthy or happy. But if you want to shake things up a bit, my advice is to try at least a few of these steps and watch what happens.

1. **Discuss your plan with your significant other.** Let your partner know that he may be getting a few surprises, and that it's going to be a time for experimentation. Tell him that it will be like an intimate vacation or second honeymoon, although you won't be leaving town. Even though you may be a little uncomfortable declaring your intentions, opening up communications on the subject of sex is an important step in improving this area of your life. Remember that this is a partnership; this is something that you want to do to improve your partner's sex life as well as your own. Get your partner involved in planning some of the fun. What man isn't going to be excited by the thought of having more sex?

2. **Start your day with a roll in the hay.** Sex in the morning is one of the best ways to keep a healthy sex life going. There are physiological and psychological reasons for this. As we learned earlier in the book, your cortisol levels start high in the morning and decline over the course of the day with intermittent rises as stressors arouse the adrenal gland. What usually happens is that you wake up, get out of bed, and are instantly thrown into the stress-producing situation of getting the kids ready for school, getting yourself ready for work, driving the car pool, figuring out who's going to drive which kid to which after-school activity, and on and on. If you get up a few minutes early to have sex with your spouse (and let's face it, it will probably take only a few minutes), you keep the cortisol levels high a bit longer, and then it gradually drops without having the huge peaks and valleys that are the usual morning fare. Additionally, sex produces endorphins, the body's feel-good hormones (see page 130 for a longer explanation), which help give you an energy boost and stabilize your mood for the rest of the day. And then when you're exhausted at night, perhaps your partner won't be so insistent.

3. **Add some variety to your life.** Sex in the morning may not always be possible. What about a little afternoon delight? Perhaps you and your mate can both arrange to come home

for lunch while the kids are in school. If you have kids, sneak off into the garage, and do it in the back seat of the car for 10 or 15 minutes while the kids are being supervised elsewhere. Do it in the closet, or the bathroom, or the shower. If your husband has a lockable office, maybe you can bring him an after-hours snack when everyone else has left the building. Then when your spouse returns to his office the following day, he'll be thinking about what happened the night before. Remember that being sexual doesn't always have to mean having intercourse; it can be oral sex or even just fondling. It's the surprise and variety that adds so much to the quality of the relationship.

4. **Learn to please yourself.** If you want to get in the mood, rediscover what makes you feel good. Do it by yourself (we all know what "it" means, don't we?), do it before your husband gets there, or do it with your husband. Wear something sexy to bed whether your partner is there or not. (Have you seen what most women wear to bed?) Or wear nothing at all—although most men find a bit of silky underwear sexier than a completely nude body. Educate (or remind) your partner what you like, and ask him to do the same for you. Have fun with it. Remember that we, as primates, are one of the few animals that can have multiple orgasms. Take advantage of that fact, especially if you don't have a partner at the moment. Single women certainly deserve the health and energy benefits of a great sex life as much as those who are in committed relationships. (Despite what you may think, married women statistically have more sex than single women. According to *The Case for Marriage* by Linda J. Waite and Maggie Gallagher, 43 percent of married people have sex twice a week as compared to 20 to 26 percent of single and cohabitating men and women.) Married or single, more women than ever before are taking time to pleasure themselves. A 2008 survey quizzed more than 1,000 women in the UK aged 18 to 30 to find out about their sexual attitudes and habits. The results showed that practices have certainly changed over the years: 92 percent of women admitted to masturbating, as opposed to 74 percent in 1979 and 62 percent in 1953.

5. **Don't take your work to bed.** The bedroom is for two things and two things only: sex and sleep. Put your laptop away. Lock your papers in your briefcase. Turn off the TV. If you condition yourself that this is the way it is supposed to be, you won't need those other distractions.

6. **Give yourself a chocolate treat.** Chocolate has long been known as a sensual treat, and it has some scientific backing. The rush of endorphins produced by eating chocolates, particularly dark chocolates, is similar to the pleasurable feelings associated with a healthy sexual relationship. Chocolate also contains phenylethylamine which is known to stimulate the release of dopamine into the pleasure centers commonly associated with an orgasm. I recommend trying an extra-special chocolate treat called K Sensual, bite-sized chocolate pieces infused with a combination of ancient Chinese herbs (including one called *horny goat weed*) meant to temporarily increase a woman's sensitivity. Take one chocolate with either a warm drink or an alcoholic beverage at lunchtime and another with a warm drink or an alcoholic beverage just before intended intimacy (you can find this product at www.dianekronchocolates.com).

7. **Make sex a priority.** Some couples put aside a date night once a week, but that doesn't necessarily translate into having sex. So if your sex life isn't quite what you want it to be, you have to plan intimacy. There's an old saying that goes "fail to plan, plan to fail." Ask yourself this question: *Is sex a luxury or a necessity?* For most couples, it is essential to the health of their relationship. Start setting aside some time each week when you plan sex, and then make sure you carry out your plan. This will help you get back into the swing of sex and make it a pleasurable part of your life's routine.

In this chapter you've learned the dos and don'ts for an active and pleasurable sex life at any age. We've covered the ways to upgrade your hormonal balance and enhance your well-being and libido. I encourage you to try new things and get your groove back, be playful and willing to listen to your partner's needs as well as speak up for your own. Lovemaking is more than an instinctual desire; it's an opportunity for caring, comfort, and a vital component to every woman's life. Now it's time to get your body moving outside of the bedroom to boost your metabolism and keep that good energy flowing.

CHAPTER 6

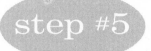

Move Your Body and Boost Your Metabolism

Here's my basic philosophy about exercise: no excuses. I've been an athlete (or at least athletic) for most of my life; I was on my high-school ski team and, until recently, continued to ski throughout my adult life. Then . . . during the course of writing this book, I had three surgeries for injuries incurred while enjoying the sport I love so much. I thought, *What do I do now?* I could just stop my athletics. Who could blame me? I've got a really good excuse. I could say my knees and ankles are done, and that's that. But I'm not so easily defeated.

I tried cross-country skiing, but I didn't get the adrenaline rush I got with downhill skiing. I tried snow shoeing. The only one who enjoyed going with me was my dog, but the snow was too deep for him, and he couldn't handle it. So I decided to take up snowboarding. I'm considered middle aged and I took up a radical sport that I never in my life wanted to do—that I had *no interest* in doing—but I'm doing it. And it's hard. But I'm doing it. I'm in pain, but I'm doing it.

I can't tell you how many times a patient who in the past had been successful at losing weight, had been eating healthily, and had exercised routinely, enters my office having gained several pounds since their last visit. They justify their extra pounds by explaining that they can no longer exercise because they got into a car accident or they fell off the curb and sprained their back, or . . . something came up that disrupted their routine and they can't do what they used to do.

I don't let them get away with it. You broke your ankle? Work your upper body. You had knee surgery? Do sit-ups. Unless you're in a full-body cast, there is probably some way you can find to get the rest of your body moving.

When I decided to take up snowboarding, the first thing I did was go online and order equipment. Then I took my first lesson. Sounds like I did things backward, but I know myself all too well, and it actually made perfect sense. My first lesson was a disaster. Frankly, I would have preferred being in a boxing ring with a heavyweight champ to doing that first day over again. I was miserable. The only reason I didn't quit right then and there was because I was already financially invested in it. That's why I bought the equipment first. It would have been too easy to give up, to find an excuse. But I had my board staring me in the face. My second lesson was so bad that my instructor gave me my money back for the lesson. Ah, but the third lesson . . . well, let's say I'm officially a snowboarder now, and getting the most amazing workout of my life. The point is I didn't let my injuries become an excuse. If you face a barrier, you find a way to get over it, under it, or around it. You recreate yourself. You do something else.

TOO TIRED TO EXERCISE? EXERCISE MORE.

I know. You're tired. That's why you're reading this book. You've been putting off reading this chapter (you may even have considered skipping it altogether) because, let's face it, you don't really want to exercise. You don't really want to get out of bed or up off the couch. That old inertia principle has got you in its spell: a body at rest tends to stay at rest. It takes so much *energy* to get yourself moving. Just the thought of exercising is simply exhausting.

Personally, I don't usually feel that way. I've trekked all over the world, hiked hundreds of trails, and climbed several mountains.

Even so, there have been times when I've been so busy living my everyday hectic life as a doctor, wife, and mother that I just can't bear the thought of getting up early to exercise when I'd so much rather sleep in for another half hour.

Here is what has convinced me to get up and get moving: scientists have concluded that one of the best ways to beat fatigue and boost energy is to exercise more, not less. Studies have shown that the more you move—and it doesn't have to be major movement, just getting up and walking around the room will help—the more energy you will feel. In fact, a 2008 study published in the journal *Psychotherapy and Psychosomatics* reported that inactive people who normally complained of fatigue could increase energy by 20 percent and decrease fatigue by as much as 65 percent by simply participating in regular, low-intensity exercise. Other studies have shown that you can increase more energy and reduce more fatigue through exercise than by using stimulant medications, and that this applied across the board to every group that was studied, including healthy adults, cancer patients, and people with diabetes and heart disease.

The explanation for this goes deep into the cellular level of the body, where we find the mitochondria, those tiny, energy-producing organs found in every cell of the body. The more you move around, the more mitochondria your body makes to meet your energy needs. The more mitochondria you have, the greater the boost to your metabolism, and the greater your ability to produce more energy.

As we learned in the detox chapter, getting rid of toxins in the body will give you more energy. So here's another reason to exercise: exercise accelerates the detoxification process. Exercise pushes the blood to circulate more efficiently through the body, allowing nutrients to more easily reach all the organs and muscles. At the same time, exercise helps lymph fluids circulate through the body, which removes toxins and other harmful materials. When you exercise, you naturally take in more oxygen; to make room for the added oxygen, your cells kick out toxins that are taking up space. When you exercise properly, you build up a sweat and toxins are released through the pores of the skin.

Of course, exercise does more than give you more energy. Exercise also reduces the risk for heart disease and stroke, high blood pressure, diabetes, obesity, back pain, osteoporosis, breast cancer, and colon cancer. It improves your cholesterol and boosts your immune system. When you exercise, your muscles use glucose for energy, reducing your blood glucose levels. It helps you sleep better. It causes the body to release endorphins that can help relieve stress and depression, and pump up the volume on feelings of peace and happiness. Exercise also releases adrenaline, serotonin, and dopamine, all of which work together as natural mood and energy boosters.

START WITH BABY STEPS

If you think about human beings and the way we are made, you begin to realize that it goes against our human nature, not to mention our human biology, to be sedentary. We are not built to sit behind a desk. We began as hunters. We weren't even gatherers or farmers until much later in our evolution. Our ancestors spent their lives being chased by animals that were trying to eat them and chasing animals they were trying to eat. It was never necessary to think about exercise as something separate from what you did all day, which was chase and be chased. Thousands of years later, our bodies have not changed very much, but our attitude toward movement has. We may spend the day chasing after a new client or account, but we don't even have to get off our behinds to do that. Our fingers get more exercise typing and texting than the whole rest of our bodies. For many of us, exercise has become another difficult chore that has to be fit in somewhere between the babies and the boardroom. Sometimes it takes more of an attitude adjustment than anything else to get yourself going on an exercise routine, especially if you lead a sedentary life and haven't exercised in a while (if ever). My advice as to the best way to get going? One baby step at a time.

This may seem contradictory to the "no excuses" philosophy I talked about earlier, but it's not. I also believe in being realistic.

I understand that many of us are all-or-nothing people. We dive headlong into the pool or we don't go in at all. We join a gym, go every day for a month, puff away on the treadmill or the elliptical, and then, when it gets too hard to keep up the pace, we quit. Our bodies can't keep up with our good intentions. If you need to lose weight and haven't exercised in a while, don't jump into a training regimen right away. Start your nutrition program first, lose a few pounds, and then begin your exercise program. If you're 80 pounds overweight and you go to the gym, you're going to get discouraged when you can't go more than three minutes at a time without losing your breath. A 2009 study from the Netherlands showed that starting and staying with a serious exercise program is much easier *after* you've lost some weight. It's not that overweight people are lazy or unwilling. It's just that exercise is much more difficult if you're carrying around extra pounds.

Most people give up when they don't see results right away. We are a culture of instant gratification. If we try hard for a few days and don't see results, it's easy for us to quit. It can also be intimidating or embarrassing to go to a gym where everyone else seems to be in much better shape. In that case, you may be better off starting an exercise program at home or going to a gym that caters specifically to women. When you start to lose weight first, you'll feel lighter and have more stamina. Get your nutrition together, get your sleep patterns in order, get your sexual energy in place, start taking your recommended supplements, and then it will be much easier to begin your exercise program.

From Dr. Eva's Files

Maryellen was 60 years old, overweight, and had recently lost her mother. She was exhausted, and her eating was out of control. She came to me to help her lose weight. We discussed nutrition for a while and then I asked her about her level of exercise. She said she was a pretty sedentary person. "But," she said, "I'm going to join a gym on Monday."

"You're 60 years old, and you've never joined a gym before, have you?"

"No," she said.

"So what makes you think you're going to join a gym now?" I asked.

She looked embarrassed and admitted that the chances of her going to the gym if she did actually join were slim to none. "I do have a treadmill at home," she said cheerily.

"Do you use it?" No again.

"If you don't use your treadmill at home, are you really going to go the gym and use one there?"

"I guess not," she said.

I suggested she put the gym on the back burner for the time being, concentrate on changing her diet first, and slowly begin walking more and working out to a beginner-level home exercise tape.

She came back to me two months later, having lost 20 pounds. Not only that, a week earlier she had suddenly felt ready to start using the treadmill. She'd been on it several times already, and was now making it part of her morning routine.

"It made so much sense for me to wait," she said. "Now I feel like I have the energy to use the treadmill and it makes me feel great for the rest of the day."

Once you begin an exercise program, you're best off starting with baby steps. Jason Muirbrook, a Los Angeles–based former model and certified personal trainer with a roster of A-list clients, tells the story of a 300-plus-pound female client of his who wanted to lose weight but was having difficulty finding exercises she could actually do. He recommended that she sit on the edge of her bed every morning and simply stand up and sit down 20 times. This was something she could do on her own without feeling overwhelmed. She started with 20 repetitions, worked her way up to 100 and lost 23 pounds, which then gave her the ability and the confidence to start incorporating more traditional exercises into her program. Throwing people into a fitness regime is a set-up for failure, says Muirbrook. "You don't change your habits or your body overnight. Giving yourself a huge goal, like 'I'm going to lose 100 pounds' is often too daunting to be realistic. What works is to take it one day at a time. It takes time, whether it's having a soda addict start by eliminating one can a day, or asking an obese person to add in one simple exercise. The results will follow, which makes it easier to take the next step to a healthier lifestyle."

In fact, you can get some of the benefits of exercise just by fidgeting. Researchers at the Mayo Clinic examined the role of nonexercise activity thermogenesis—calories burned during the activities of daily living—and found that thin people incorporate more spurts of activity, such as fidgeting, into their daily lives than their heavier counterparts. They suggest that you can add more energy to your life by adding little bursts of activity to your day: delivering a message to your colleague at work in person rather than by e-mail, standing more often (rather than being a constant couch potato), walking around the room, and even tapping your toes when watching TV.

Be Honest with Yourself

If you want to get more energy out of exercising, you have to put your heart into it. Literally. Although fidgeting and walking around the room may help you get started on the right track, these tips are just that: a way to get started. Wiggling your toes isn't going to produce very many new energized mitochondria. If you want to get results, you have to keep working your way up to new energy levels.

One phenomenon I see all the time is patients who are fooling themselves. I ask them if they work out and they swear they do. But their definition of working out isn't necessarily the same as mine. There is one patient with whom I have the same conversation year after year. As she has aged, she has gained weight around her middle, and she is concerned about diabetes, which runs in her family. She comes in annually to have blood work done. Her test results tell me she is on her way to the disease, and her results are getting worse every time. When I ask her if she is working out, she says that she is, but even her tone tells me she is not quite telling the truth. "Oh," she says, "I get on my stationary bike for a while and then I lift some weights." When I try to pin her down on her definition of "a while," she tells me it changes every day because of her busy schedule. Every visit I tell her she needs to do more, but every visit she comes back with the same description of her routine. I believe that she believes she is exercising, but she is, in fact, fooling herself.

There are some people who love to exercise, who are addicted to exercise. I want to make it very clear: I am not one of those people. I do it because I know I have to do it. Every day that I make an appointment with myself to do one activity or another, I have to negotiate with myself. Usually my better judgment prevails and I go through with it. I exercise because I want to keep my body as healthy as possible for as long as possible. I never want to say that I can't do something or travel somewhere because I don't have the strength or because I'm too tired or out of shape. I've traveled around the world with people in their 70s and 80s who endure like 20-year-olds, and it's because they keep active and have been active all their lives. I do what I have to do to be like them.

But I'm not perfect. More than once I have been guilty of the "bargain maneuver." I remember one day in particular when I got up at 6:00 in the morning and dragged myself downstairs to my stationary bike, which I had planned to ride for 30 minutes. After 15 minutes, I started negotiating with myself. Not because I was feeling the burn or was out of breath, but just because I was bored. *I'll only do 20 minutes today,* I told myself, *because I'll be running around all day, and I'll burn off the calories. And I'll do 10 more minutes on the bike when I get home after work.* As I'm sure you can guess, I had a very busy day at the office and didn't get in half the running around I thought I would. And because I was so tired when I got home, I had dinner, watched a little TV, and went to bed. I convinced myself, despite everything I know about exercise and all the advice I give my patients, that those ten minutes didn't matter anyway.

We all know those minutes do matter. Since that day, I have tried to be more honest with myself. If I set aside 30 minutes to exercise, I exercise for 30 minutes, and I urge my patients to do the same. Make a commitment and follow through. The result is more energy, plus it does wonders for your sense of self-esteem and accomplishment.

WHAT TYPE OF EXERCISE IS BEST FOR ENERGY?

The simplest answer to this question is the exercise that you will do. The most important thing is to get your body moving. If you sign up for a spin class and then never go, it does you no good. There are many types of exercise from which to choose and all of them give you energy to one extent or another, no doubt about it. Most exercises fit into one of three categories:

- ❖ **Aerobic exercise:** This type of exercise is the most obvious energy-producer. Plus it's heart-healthy, helps your lungs function more efficiently, and increases overall energy. Aerobic exercise is any type of exercise that gets the heart pumping and promotes the circulation of oxygen through the blood.

- ❖ **Resistance exercise:** Also referred to as strength training, resistence exercise builds muscle mass and boosts your metabolism, which in turn increases energy. Strength training also reduces blood sugar. Muscle mass stores excess blood sugar in the form of glycogen. We lose muscle mass as we age, which means we lose some of our capacity to store glucose. Too much glucose in the blood can lead to diabetes. As you build up muscle, you decrease the amount of glucose in the blood. Muscle also burns more energy when a person is at rest than fat does, so building your muscles will help you burn more calories, maintain a healthy weight, and increase your energy reserves.

❖ **Flexibility exercise:** Exercises such as yoga and tai chi are stress relievers—and we all know that stress is an energy sapper. This type of exercise focuses on stretching and breathing. The practice of yoga helps people to restore their levels of energy, to enhance stamina, relieve anxiety, and reduce fatigue. It gives you a sense of peace, which then allows you to sleep, which in turn gives you energy. Many forms of yoga focus on the art of reviving tired muscles and bringing them back to their energized state. People who are more flexible also sustain fewer injuries.

The best way to increase and maintain energy is to include all three types.

The Ancient Art of Tai Chi

When my family and I were traveling by boat on the Yangtze River in China, we were awakened every morning not by a buzzing alarm clock but by elegant music chiming in the background. It was a very relaxing way to wake up, and I knew it was something I would miss when we disembarked. Much to my surprise, as we traveled to various cities throughout China, I continued to wake up just after dawn to these melodious sounds. What I finally discovered was that I was hearing the music accompanying thousands of people practicing tai chi on the streets and in the parks to start their day.

Tai chi started out as one of the Chinese martial arts, but today is primarily practiced for its health benefits. It emphasizes complete relaxation and has been called "meditation in motion." It is characterized by soft, slow, flowing movements that are executed precisely; each posture flows seamlessly into the next without pausing, ensuring that your body is in constant motion.

Chi is an ancient Chinese notion designating a form of energy. According to the philosophy of tai chi, this energy, or chi, flows throughout the body but can become blocked, at which point one suffers from some form of illness. Tai chi is one method the Chinese use to free up the flow of chi (acupuncture is another method). Tai chi is an effective way to decrease stress, improve balance and coordination, and increase energy, endurance, and agility.

Many people in the West enjoy tai chi because it is relatively easy to learn, requires no special equipment, can be practiced indoors or outdoors, and can be done either alone or in a group. You can find tai chi classes in many communities today, including places such as the YMCA, health clubs, senior centers, and community education centers.

Experiment with Different Types of Training

There are many different ways of exercising. If you find a type that excites you and motivates you to keep exercising, that's the one you should do. But there are three types that are particularly good for increasing energy: burst training, interval training, and velocity training.

❖ **Practice Burst Training:** Burst training can strengthen your adrenal glands and prevent adrenal fatigue. Burst sessions work out the aerobic as well as anaerobic energy production in the body:

- Exercise at 90 percent of your maximum effort for 30 to 60 seconds. (This puts you in sugar-burning mode, the opposite of traditional aerobic training.) You can do this a number of ways: running fast, running/walking uphill, running up stairs, sprinting on a bicycle, treadmill, elliptical, Stairmaster, etc. You should feel like it's going to kill you, but you never do it for more than 60 seconds.

- Next, rest for 60 to 120 seconds. Your recovery time should be twice as long as your exercise time, so if you exercised for 60 seconds, your recovery time is 120 seconds. (Do *nothing* except catch your breath.)

- ◆ Repeat steps one and two.

- ◆ You should do this so that your total burst-exercise time is 7 to 9 minutes, 4 days a week.

Burst training causes your body to burn fat for the next 36 hours to replace your body's vital energy (glycogen) stores. It also increases the efficiency of how well your muscles draw oxygen from your blood. This is also known as oxygen uptake. When this happens, your muscles have more energy to work longer, harder, and healthier. You want to build up as much lactic acid as you can (an organic acid produced in mammals during the breakdown of glucose when oxygen is in short supply); lactic acid then increases growth hormone and testosterone. In essence, it increases metabolism. You want to recover twice as long so you can diffuse the discomfort that lactic acid produces. You've probably done burst training without even realizing it by sprinting across a parking lot to avoid a downpour or running to catch a bus.

❖ **Interval training:** Interval training is somewhat akin to burst training. It's one of the fastest ways to create a body that is faster, stronger, and healthier—not to more energetic. In this type of workout, you increase the intensity or pace for several minutes, then back off for anywhere from two to ten minutes (depending on how long your total workout will be, and how much time you need to recover). High intensity usually means that you're working at anywhere from 70 to 85 percent of your maximum heart rate. You can calculate your maximum heart rate by subtracting your age from 220. In burst training you do nothing during the rest period, but in interval training you keep moving but lower the intensity. It's as if you were taking a brisk walk on a very hilly trail. Going up a high hill at a brisk pace will raise your heartbeat and make your muscles work harder. On the way down the hill, you're still moving, but at a much lower intensity. Many treadmills offer the option of programming in interval training so that it automatically goes faster and slower and changes the incline. Your metabolic response will be much greater than when you're doing the normal boring walking (or even running) on the treadmill. If you go at the same fixed pace and always do the same workout, your body gets so comfortable that it's not challenged anymore, and it will not help you increase your energy. You can do interval training with any kind of activity, including walking, running, swimming, cycling, dancing, jumping rope, etc.

❖ **Velocity training:** This workout will include what my physical therapist, whom I went to see following a skiing injury, calls velocity training. It's a kind of strength training that concentrates on balance—it's a burst of energy while holding your body is in a specific muscular motion. Here's one example: You lay a rope (or a resistance band) on the floor in the middle of the room. Starting at one end of the rope, you jump with both legs over the rope, moving forward with each jump until you reach the other end. You then jump backward over the rope until you reach your starting position again. Another exercise is to set up two chairs on either side of the room with a clear space in between them. Keeping your knees bent, you sprint sideways back and forth between the two chairs. These types of exercises can be done at home, take a short amount of time, and give you the energy boost you need to get through the day.

A New Type of Training

Believe it or not, there was a time when there was no such thing as a treadmill or an elliptical machine—or any other kind of exercise machine, for that matter. Times have certainly changed, and new kinds of mechanical exercise aids are being introduced every day. One of the newest is called the Power Plate, and it's something I personally have found very effective. A study presented at the 2009 European Congress on Obesity found that overweight or obese people who regularly used exercise equipment in combination with a calorie-restricted diet were more successful at long-term weight loss and shedding fat around their abdominal organs than those who combined dieting with a more conventional fitness routine. The Power Plate machine consists of a vibrating base, which may vibrate up and down approximately 1/16 of an inch 25 to 50 times per second. According to Power Plate's manufacturers, if you stand on the machine's vibrating plates for 10 minutes a day three times a week, you will lose weight, increase bone density and improve your overall health. The Power Plate uses whole-body vibration, or WBV, to contract muscles 30 to 50 times per second. The continual vibration causes you to tense and relax your muscles to keep your balance. But to get the most out of the Power Plate, you perform exercises you already know while on the machine, such as squats, triceps dips, and push-ups. The motion makes the exercise positions harder to hold. It looks like it is a lazy person's way out, but that's not the case at all. The Power Plate is not a magic bullet. In order for it to be most effective, you need to use the machine in combination with a healthy diet and aerobic exercise.

Find a Sport You Love

One of the best ways to get motivated to exercise is to participate in a sport. It's not just about energy. It's not just about getting in shape. It's about achieving a goal—to be good at whatever sport you choose, whether it's rollerblading, swimming, playing tennis, or beach volley ball. It doesn't matter what sport it is, it only matters that you enjoy it. If you start young, you won't spend so much time in front of the computer or the television. Having said that, you're never too old to start a new sport. The feeling of accomplishment you get simply by participating actually increases your energy output. Many of my patients who are fatigued have discovered dancing (a variation on the "sport" concept). One of the reasons they find it so appealing is that there are so many kinds of dance and dance classes available. Some go to ballroom or swing dance classes; others go to classes that are closer to exercise classes and don't require partners. If you prefer not going to a class, you can dance around the house or arrange a "dance night" with friends and neighbors.

From Dr. Eva's Files

As I was speaking to one of my patients about her exercise routine, she told me that she did not like the thought of going to a gym. She would rather, she said, find alternatives to treadmills and gym equipment.

"It's very difficult for some people like me, especially when you get into your 50s or 60s, to join a gym," Cecile told me. "You're not prepared for the invasion of your privacy, especially in the locker room. There's no private space, and you have to share a space with everyone. It's like walking into a nudist colony for the first time: you find yourself feeling awkward and imagine that all eyes are on you. Some people in the gym are very aggressive; they're very focused. They sometimes even bump into you. And if you're not prepared for that, it can be very alienating and can have a countereffect to you wanting to work out. It can be very challenging.

"In the Latin culture, we're not predisposed to exercise or a routine. Perspiring is not something we do in a communal environment. It's something very private. As women, we're not socialized to believe that we have to work out, because we're more curvaceous. It doesn't mean that we're lilies of the vine and we're supposed to be those pretty little things; it is just not in our social makeup. The only time you're sweating and letting it go is when you're dancing. That is very much a part of our culture.

"Personally, I go to a dance class three times a week. During the week I drive an hour and ten minutes to get there in traffic, but it is my escape. It's inside of a gym, but I walk through the gym, upstairs to the class, take a shower afterward, and go home. There are people in the class who are 20 and people who are 70. We feel we are part of a community. It's my release. I joke and say it's cheaper than therapy. I get to work out and stay in shape, but also I get to connect to something that is very fundamentally important to me. If I didn't do that dance class, I probably wouldn't get any exercise at all.

"It's part of what I now do to take care of myself, part of my personal Fatigue Solution program. And I know it's not an overnight fix. It took me years of ignoring my stress to get my body into horrible shape—why would I think it's going to take a month to get it into better shape? How could I be that uncaring to myself? If you're not really prepared to take responsibility, to realize that this is a lifestyle and that you have to be good to your body every day, then you are missing the true enjoyment that life gives you.

"I am replacing all my bad habits with energy and love so that I can be healthy again. Not just for a year but for the rest of my life. It's not the house you live in; it's not the car you're driving; it's not the clothes you're wearing. It is your body. It is your life."

If time is an issue (and it almost always is), there are sports you can do at home. I, for instance, have recently taken up boxing. You don't need a partner. You can use a punching bag or a video version or even a Wii. Any way you choose, it's great exercise. You only spar for three minutes at a time—go four rounds and you're done! Even my kids love it. And there's something about putting on those gloves and punching away that makes me feel sexy. And it's not just me. My husband loves to see me all messy and sweaty. It gets both our juices going . . . and that's always a good way to boost your energy (and your libido).

There are plenty of ways you can get exercise at home with minimum equipment, or none at all. You can practice burst or interval training by simply marching in place at varying speeds. You can jump rope. And you can put on your favorite music and dance around the room with nobody watching and no one giving out scores. I can't say it enough—the most important thing is to get yourself moving.

Stop the Crunches!

What's the one exercise everyone seems to love, the one you see everyone doing at the gym, and the one you're most likely to do at home? Crunches. You know, where you're down on the floor on your back and you bend your knees and place your hands behind your head and then slowly contract your abdominal muscles. However popular they may be, crunches are not the best type of exercise you can do to increase your energy levels. For one thing, most people do them incorrectly, putting an unhealthy strain on the back at its weakest point and also an unhealthy strain on the neck. In other words, you may end up creating poor posture and lower-back pain. You have to get up and move your body if you want the fat to melt away and if you want to give yourself an energy boost.

Don't Forget to Breathe

At age 36 and 30 pounds overweight, Keisha came to see me complaining that she just couldn't get rid of those extra pounds ,no matter what she did. When I asked her about exercise, she told me that she's tried many different types of exercise—running, bicycling, spinning, Zumba (a combination dance and fitness program)—but she could never last beyond the first ten minutes. I took out my stethoscope and checked her lungs. They sounded clear and strong, as did her heart. So I asked her if she wouldn't mind running in place for a minute or so right in my office to see if I could detect any problems. She agreed. As she began to run, the diagnosis quickly became apparent. Keisha kept forgetting to breathe! And when she did, she wasn't breathing from her diaphragm. No wonder she couldn't exercise for more than a few minutes. I pointed this out to her and suggested that she work with a personal trainer for a few sessions so that the trainer could teach her the proper way to breathe.

Breathing is something we don't think about very much because it's automatic, but it is actually a very important component of any exercise routine. If you have nothing to drink, you can survive for several days. If you have nothing to eat, you can survive for several weeks. But if you don't have oxygen, you can't survive for more than a few minutes. One of the most common mistakes people make while exercising is that they don't breathe correctly or they don't breathe at all. This can be the source of fatigue and overexertion. And this can result in shortness of breath and a painful stitch in your side, which can cause you to stop exercising all together. And worse, it can cause your blood pressure to rise.

When you breathe correctly, you get enough oxygen in your system to increase your circulation and get the blood flowing to every part of your body, including the brain. That makes it easier for the brain to release the neurotransmitters that boost both your mood and your energy. If you're breathing properly during exercise, you will probably make an audible grunting or whooshing noise as you breathe in and out.

Here are some tips to keep breathing properly during your exercise routine (whichever type of exercise you choose):

❖ Start with a warm up—you can warm up your breathing techniques at the same time you're getting your muscles ready for a workout. Take a few minutes to simply inhale and exhale and focus on your breathing.

❖ Inhale through your nose, fill up your lungs, and exhale slowly through your mouth. Exhaling should take roughly twice as long as inhaling.

❖ Breathe in on the exertion part of the exercise. For instance, if you are doing a squat, breathe in when you are bending your legs and moving downward, and breathe out when you are standing up again. This can help lower blood pressure and cortisol levels while supplying oxygen to the muscles.

❖ Never hold your breath during exercise. This can cause your blood pressure to shoot up and lead to dizziness and fatigue.

❖ Listen to your body. Don't let yourself get to the point where you're hyperventilating or gasping for air. That means you're working way too hard and you need to slow down and catch your breath.

DRESS FOR WORKOUT SUCCESS

No, this isn't a fashion statement. Despite what some gyms may make you feel, how you look when you exercise doesn't make a bit of difference. The most important factor is that what you wear is comfortable and supports anything that needs to be supported. I've heard ridiculous stories from patients who were wearing the wrong things and paid the price for it. For instance, one patient of mine went to New York for a weekend of sightseeing and the only shoes she brought were flip-flops. Needless to say, her feet were killing her by the time she got home to Los Angeles. I've even known women who have gone hiking in heels. They were lucky they did not do permanent damage to themselves.

Here are some tips for your workout gear:

❖ **Not all shoes are alike.** The type of exercise you're primarily doing determines what type of shoe you need. If you like aerobics, step, kickboxing, and other high-impact workouts, you need a shoe with good shock absorption and stability. If you're more into strength training and cardio equipment with an occasional foray into other activities such as walking, try a cross-trainer that is lightweight, durable, and offers moderate cushioning and stability. If you're a more athletic girl and you enjoy running and jumping type of exercising, you need a running shoe that supports explosive heavy pounding and stop-start activity. If you enjoy walking, hiking, biking, and other outdoor activities, you probably need a walking shoe with excellent ankle support. The newest innovation in sports footwear is toning shoes, made with a deliberately unstable surface. The instability forces wearers to activate muscles they would not use otherwise, as they work to align and balance the body with each step. As a result, women who wear toning shoes expend more energy and produce greater effort to walk than if they were wearing traditional shoes. You might want to shop for any type of sports shoes in stores that specialize in athletic wear because they usually have staff who can advise you on which type of shoe you need for the exercise you choose.

❖ **Wear cotton.** If you exercise in spandex, you may end up with a yeast infection or candidiasis, which as we know is a definite energy depleter.

❖ **Don't wear a thong.** I know this is gross, but a thong can pull feces into your vagina if you're doing a lot of back and forth motions, and that can give you a urinary tract infection. It can also cause bacterial vaginosis, which is a disruption of the normal flora that lives in the vaginal area. My suggestion? Although wearing a thong may rid you of those ugly panty lines (even more evident when you're wearing tight exercise gear), lose the thong. You're better off wearing *no* underwear than a thong.

❖ **Wear a good bra.** Finding the right sports bra takes trial and error. It all depends on what size you are and what type of exercise you normally practice. Sports bras are specially designed to help minimize movement during your workout and offer better support and more comfort than a regular bra. Along with the fatty tissue and mammary glands that are in your breasts, ligaments help keep the breasts firm and perky. Exercising in the wrong bra can stretch these ligaments, leading to greater sagging and even pain during exercise.

TIMING IS EVERYTHING

I'm one of those people who prefers to get up early and exercise before I officially start my day. It not only gets me going, energy-wise, for the rest of the day, it also gives me peace of mind knowing that I've gotten that "obligation" over with. And I don't have to worry about unforeseen circumstances arising during the day that might squeeze out my exercise time. Other people prefer to work out during their lunch break or to go to the gym directly after work. I've even known a few die-hards who will get on the treadmill at midnight if they can't find any other time in the day.

Is there a perfect time to exercise? According to our bodies' cycles, adrenal hormones are highest in the morning, then slowly decrease to their lowest point, which is when we're ready for bed. What happens when we exercise late in the day? We throw off the cycle, as exercise stimulates the adrenal gland. You end up with a burst of energy into the night, resulting in insomnia. Exercising at night (as well as eating too late in the evening) raises your heart rate and body temperature, which makes it difficult to fall asleep. I recommend that you finish your exercising before 4:00 P.M. if at all possible.

Exercising early doesn't always fit into your schedule. And people who are more night owls than early birds many find it difficult to get going in the morning and would rather have more sleep time. I have several patients who find it much easier to exercise right after work when they are already out and about. If that's what works best for you, then I say go for it. Just be sure to find ways to calm yourself down before bedtime—do some inspirational reading, listen to soothing music, do a few yoga stretches—that will allow your body to fall asleep.

You don't need to exercise for hours at a time (in fact, you shouldn't). Each exercise session should last for no more than 45 minutes to an hour or your body starts to go into exhaustion mode. Even if you only exercise for a short period of time, your mood will be improved. Just ten minutes of moderate exercise is enough to improve your mood, your vigor, and decrease fatigue. However, to obtain all the benefits from exercise, not just the mood-improving aspects, you should do at least 30 minutes of moderate exercise every day. To get the most benefit, alternate the types of exercises you do. For instance, you might try burst training on Monday, brisk walking on Tuesday, interval training on Wednesday, burst training on Thursday, and so on, with perhaps one day with no exercise at all. Once your body is acclimated to exercising, you can work out every other day, increasing and intensifying your routine as you get stronger.

What matters most, however, is that you find a time of day that is consistently good for you. That way, exercise can become a part of your regular routine, just like brushing your teeth. People who exercise at random times during the day, especially people who are just starting to get themselves moving, are more likely to drop out. Once you establish exercise as a habit, it's much easier to keep it going.

THE BOOST YOUR METABOLISM
jump-start tips

The most important concept you can learn about exercise, according to trainer Jason Muirbrook, is that of the "metabolic shock." The best exercises you can do for energy are multijoint exercises because they use more than one motion, causing your body to exert such an effort that it throws you into a state of metabolic shock. This metabolic shock actually causes you to burn more calories for long after the workout is over. That's why you start slowly and build your way up. Every time you change your routine or increase the number of reps you do, you disturb your system and force it to develop more energy.

Now that we know a little about how exercise and energy are connected, there are specific exercises that are good for increasing energy and some that are not so good. Walking, for instance, has many benefits: it's good for your heart and your bones and your muscles, but not necessarily for increasing energy. The problem is that in order for exercise to increase your energy, it has to increase your heart rate. Many doctors recommend a brisk walk—meaning a walk that raises your pulse rate to 160. But can you sustain that for 20 minutes? Most people can't keep up the pace. Even when they intend to go out for a brisk walk it usually turns out to be more like a casual stroll.

Here are some energy-enhancing exercises, provided by Jason Muirbrook, that you can do at home and incorporate into a regular exercise routine:

❖ **Squats:** Start with your feet on the floor, shoulder-width apart, your back straight and your core engaged (by drawing your belly button in and slightly up). Once in position, slowly bend your knees and lower your hips toward the floor, keeping your torso straight and your knees behind your toes and pointed directly front. The objective is to keep your thighs parallel to the floor and hold for a few seconds. Your feet should be firmly on the floor, not in the air. Once you have gone down to about 90 degrees at the knees, stand back up to the starting position and repeat. If you are a beginner, you can do a modified squat by sitting on a chair with your feet flat on the floor, your back straight and your core engaged. Then stand up without using your arms for support. Sit back down, again without using your arms, and repeat. Do this 25 times in a row, rest for 20 seconds, and repeat. If you feel that you can't get through that many reps, try doing 15 or 20 and work your way up to 25.

❖ **Squat and curl:** This is the same squat exercise, either standing or sitting, except that you are adding some weights. Get into your starting position while holding a lightweight dumbbell (or a filled bottle of water or a can of soup) in each hand, arms at your side, palms facing front. As you stand up after the squat, keep your elbows close to your side and curl your hands up toward your shoulders, bending at the elbow. Straighten your arms back down to your sides to the starting position and repeat.

❖ **Lunges:** Like squats, lunges work most of the muscles in your legs including your quads, hamstrings, glutes, and calves. Start with both feet flat on the floor shoulder-width apart, your back straight, and your core engaged. Take a giant step forward with your right leg, keeping the front knee and back knee at 90-degree angles. Your toes and knees should be pointing straight to the front. The back leg will bend, almost reaching the floor. Hold the position for a few seconds. Make sure not to extend your front knee past your toes because that puts a lot of stress on the joint. To keep your balance, you will have to push your weight into the heels and not the toes. Push your body back up to the starting position through your front heel. Repeat with your left leg forward. Start with ten lunges on each leg, rest for 20 seconds, and repeat.

❖ **Leg kicks:** Kneel on all fours with hands flat on the floor, in a table-like position. If you have sore knees and cannot kneel on the hard floor, fold up a towel and place it evenly underneath both knees. Keeping your back flat and your core engaged, extend your right leg straight back until it is parallel to the floor and squeeze your gluteus (butt) muscle. Hold for a few seconds and return to the starting position. Repeat using the left leg. Start with ten kicks on each leg, rest for 20 seconds, repeat.

❖ **Glute side kicks** (aka, doggie peeing on a hydrant): Start on all fours on the floor. From a kneeling position, raise your right leg keeping your thigh parallel to the floor and your knee bent at a 90-degree angle. Slowly straighten your leg, but do not lock the knee. Hold for the count of five and slowly bend the knee back to the starting position. Repeat ten times, rest for 20 seconds, and then switch to the other leg.

As you get stronger, you can increase the number of reps for each exercise and make the rest periods shorter. These are exercises you can do for 30 minutes, five days a week. They will get your muscles toned and your heartbeat racing. These can be done in conjunction with whatever cardio workout you choose to do, whether it is running on a trail or track, using the treadmill, playing a sport, or going to a spinning class.

Now that you've read these first six chapters and made the suggested environmental and lifestyle modifications, you should be well on your way to being thinner, happier, healthier, and more energized than you were before reading this book. If you're not, then you need to ask yourself this question: *Is there something biologically wrong with me?* The most common medical condition causing fatigue today is thyroid disease. Thyroid hormones are released into the bloodstream and are transported throughout the body where they control metabolism; every cell in the body depends upon thyroid hormones for regulation of their metabolism. That's why I felt it was important to devote the next chapter to the thyroid, how it works, and how to keep it working at its best for you.

CHAPTER 7

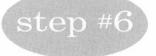

Check Your Thyroid

The woman was in her mid-50s. She had an extremely high-pressure job and was in the public eye. Her struggles with weight over the years were well known. Although most people did not know it, she had also struggled for years with symptoms such as anxiety and sleeplessness and even occasional panic attacks. In 2007, her weight gain began to escalate rapidly, and many people noticed she was looking tired all the time. Normally a high-energy type, she was now exhausted. She saw several different doctors; none of them could figure out what was wrong with her—until finally, one of them recommended thyroid testing. She started thyroid medication and within a short period of time, was feeling and looking much better. She described her diagnosis this way: "First hyperthyroidism, which sped up my metabolism and left me unable to sleep for days. (Most people lose weight. I didn't.) Then hypothyroidism, which slowed down my metabolism and made me want to sleep all the time." The woman's name is Oprah Winfrey, and until she announced her diagnosis and treatment on her famous talk show, many women in America had never even heard of the thyroid gland or thyroid disease.

If you want to see me get excited, start talking about the thyroid. Not a subject many people are passionate about, I know. But for me, this is what gets my blood boiling. Maybe it's because it's so misunderstood, so underestimated, and in so many cases, just plain ignored.

When was the last time you went to the doctor and he checked your thyroid? You would know if he did, because to manually

185

examine the thyroid, you have to step behind the patient and put your hands around the patient's neck as if you were going to choke her. That's the only way you can feel for the butterfly-shaped thyroid gland, which is located at the front of the neck near the collar bone (right where a man would wear a bowtie). When I introduce this examination to my patients, I always get the same reaction: "What are you doing? No doctor has ever done that to me before!"

That's why I say it's the gland that's ignored. You can't breathe without the thyroid, you can't think without the thyroid, you'd constantly be constipated without the thyroid, and yet it's way down at the bottom of the list of possible causes of some very common symptoms. Are you losing your hair? It could be your thyroid. Is your voice getting hoarse and raspy? It could be your thyroid. Are you always cold? It could be your thyroid. Are you having trouble concentrating? It could be your thyroid. And if it is, it's something that is easily fixed. That's why I get so angry and excited at the same time about the subject. People are suffering needlessly, some for many years, when they could be leading much more energetic, productive lives with the right diagnosis and treatment.

Those people who have heard of the thyroid usually believe it has something to do with weight loss and metabolism, and they use it as an excuse for their weight-loss difficulties. "I know I must have a thyroid problem," they'll say, "because no matter what I do, I just can't lose weight." Most of the time, that's simply not true, but it's easier to blame the thyroid than to blame their own lifestyle choices.

THE THYROID: WHAT, WHERE, AND HOW

So . . . you're reading this book because you suffer from fatigue. No surprise. You're incredibly busy, you take care of your family, you work long hours, and you have a lot of responsibilities. You try to exercise, but you don't always have time. You've been gaining weight lately, but who hasn't been? Maybe you're a bit anxious or depressed. Perhaps you're not sleeping as well as you used to, and maybe your hair is a little thinner than it was just a few months ago. A lot of women add up all these symptoms and come up with . . . nothing. It's just life; it's just getting older. But maybe, just maybe, it's more than that. Maybe it's your thyroid. In fact, one in eight women will develop a thyroid disorder during her lifetime. And by the time they reach age 60, more than 20 percent of American women will have a thyroid disorder. I personally believe the numbers may be even higher because so many women haven't been officially diagnosed.

The simplest way to describe your thyroid and its function is to compare it to a furnace that is run by a thermostat (the pituitary gland). Together, they regulate how much energy and stamina you have on a daily basis. The amount of thyroid hormone you have affects how well you sleep, how you feel when you get up in the morning, and how effectively you make it through your day.

Thyroid function affects every cell in the body. It is the main regulator of basal metabolism, which is the amount of energy needed to maintain essential physiologic functions when you are at complete rest, both physically and mentally. If your thyroid gland is not producing optimally, your cells cannot properly take in the nutrients they need, receive the right amount of oxygen, or get rid of waste materials efficiently. Thyroid hormones also affect your heart, muscles, bones, and cholesterol, to name just several of its jobs.

Introducing the 3s and 4s

There are two main hormones produced by the thyroid:

❖ Triiodothyronine, known as T_3

❖ Tetraiodothyronine, known as T_4

You may have noticed a portion of the word "iodine" in each of the hormones above. That's because the function of the thyroid gland is to take iodine, found in many foods, and convert it into thyroid hormones. Thyroid cells are the only cells in the body that can absorb iodine.

These cells combine iodine and the amino acid tyrosine to make T_3 and T_4. (Don't worry about remembering your threes and fours—I'm just trying to help you see the big picture of how the thyroid works.) The normal thyroid gland manufactures both T_3 and T_4; it produces about 80 percent T_4 and about 20 percent T_3. However, T_3 is about four times as potent as T_4. T_4 is actually a precursor to T_3. While traveling through the liver, T_4 loses one of its iodine molecules, which converts the T_4 to T_3.

There is one more factor we have to mention to complete this process, and that is thyroid stimulating hormone (TSH), which is produced by the pituitary gland in the brain and gives that gland its thermostatlike function. So the thyroid is the furnace that provides "heat" in the form of the T_3 and T_4 hormones, and the pituitary gland is the thermostat that goes on and off according to the amount of heat in the body. TSH tells the thyroid to raise or lower the heat. The process goes like this:

T_3 and T_4 travel through the bloodstream, producing heat.

The pituitary gland senses the heat; the thermostat shuts off; TSH production slows down.

The body cools as the level of thyroid hormones decrease.

The pituitary senses the decrease in temperature; the thermostat pops on; TSH production increases.

The furnace produces more heat.

When your body temperature drops, your metabolic rate drops, too. You produce less energy, and you store more calories as fat—in other words, you gain weight. You also suffer from fatigue, irritability, and the inability to concentrate. Although it is more complicated than that, what I just introduced is the bottom line.

Too Few Hormones

The most common form of thyroid disorder is hypothyroidism. Hypothyroidism occurs when the thyroid is not producing enough of its hormones. Approximately 25 million people suffer from hypothyroidism, and about half of them are undiagnosed. It is usually found in women, particularly older women. The percentage of patients with hypothyroidism is greater for women for each decade of age after age 34. That is because thyroid hormone production decreases with age.

One of the reasons that hypothyroidism often goes undiagnosed is that symptoms usually appear slowly over time, and they may appear to be signs of normal aging. Symptoms include:

- ❖ Anxiety and nightmares

- ❖ Difficulty losing weight

- ❖ Dry skin

- ❖ Easy weight gain

- ❖ Impaired concentration and memory

- ❖ Menstrual irregularities

- ❖ Mood swings

- ❖ Severe fatigue

- ❖ Thinning eyebrows

- ❖ Yellow skin from poor conversion of beta carotene to vitamin A

There are many women who have no symptoms and feel perfectly healthy, and yet, when tested, are diagnosed with hypothyroidism. These women need to be treated as well as those who have symptoms, because their slowed metabolism will result in adverse effects down the line. It's no different than having high cholesterol and not wanting to be treated because it doesn't bother you. If you're not treated for high cholesterol, you may one day have a heart attack from the accumulation of cholesterol in your arteries. If you are not treated for hypothyroidism, you may have a heart attack because of the metabolic dysfunction that your thyroid has produced over the course of many years. That's the reason testing is so important, especially as you get older and the likelihood of hypothyroidism increases.

When people hear that I am an endocrinologist, they tell me all kinds of stories. I can't tell you the number of dinners I've attended where I hear tales of women who say they'd never even heard of thyroid disease until, after years of going from one doctor to another, they were finally diagnosed and treated, and their lives were changed forever. One such story was from a woman named Cheryl, who had been suffering from ever-worsening fatigue for ten years. She would fall asleep by 8:00 P.M. every night. She never thought it was that unusual, however, because her mother had always had a very early bedtime as well. But then she started gaining weight for no reason and she just couldn't take it off—just like her mother. She started having irregular periods—but she wasn't concerned because her mother had gone through an early menopause. She was worried when she began losing handfuls of hair every month—but her mother had been wearing a wig since she was in her late 30s.

Cheryl had always been anxious about her stressful job at the university, but now her anxiety increased as her productivity decreased. After ten years of thinking these symptoms were just normal wear and tear on an aging body (although she was only in her 40s), she finally discussed her problems with her doctor. After ruling out several other possibilities, he tested her thyroid and found she had Hashimotos's thyroiditis, a disease she had never heard of.

In the United States, the most common cause of hypothyroidism is called Hashimotos's thyroiditis. This is an autoimmune disorder—in other words, the body's immune system attacks thyroid tissue. The tissue eventually becomes so inflamed that the gland can't make enough thyroid hormone. The pituitary gland, noticing the lack of these hormones, reacts by turning up the thermostat and sending out TSH to raise hormone production. But that's no longer possible because of the inflammation of the gland. Thyroid cells start to enlarge and multiply, which will eventually cause nodules and swelling.

When Cheryl told me her story at dinner, she had only been on thyroid medication for a few weeks, but she was already feeling better and said she was hopeful for the first time in a decade that she would be back to her old self again. Interestingly enough, she had forced her mother to get her thyroid tested as well and—you guessed it—her mother had hypothyroidism as well. Hashimosto's disease, like many other autoimmune diseases, is most often inherited, usually from mothers to daughters. Since her mother was in her early 60s, she had not yet been tested for thyroid disease (most doctors don't start testing their patients until they're at least 65 years old). Her mother was not pleased when she spoke to her doctor of over 30 years. When she asked him why he had never tested her thyroid, he answered, "You've always been healthy and have never spoken to me of any concerns regarding your health. We did the standard tests. Why was I to assume you had a thyroid problem?" Lesson learned: we need to rely on our doctor for guidance, but doctors are not mind readers, either. If something is bothering you, no matter how trivial or insignificant it seems, you must voice your concerns to your physician. Health is a mutual responsibility.

Too Many Hormones

When everything is functioning properly, the thyroid and pituitary work together to produce just the right amount of hormones. But there are times when the thyroid malfunctions and produces either too many or too few hormones. When the thyroid becomes overactive and produces too many hormones, you end up with a condition called hyperthyroidism. This condition affects 10 times more women than men, and usually occurs in women under 40. Here are some of the symptoms of hyperthyroidism:

❖ Being nervous, moody, weak, or tired

❖ Rapid heartbeat

❖ Excessive sweating

❖ Red, itchy skin

❖ Fine hair that is falling out

❖ Shaky hands

❖ More bowel movements than usual

❖ Shortness of breath

The most common form of this disorder is Graves' disease, which was made "famous" when first lady Barbara Bush was diagnosed with the illness in 1989 (coincidentally, her husband, President George H. W. Bush, was later diagnosed with the same disease, as was their dog, Millie). One of the stranger symptoms of Graves' disease is known as "frog eyes" where the eyeballs get pushed forward and protrude because fat builds up behind them. Graves' disease can be life threatening and can lead to heart problems if left untreated. This type of hyperthyroidism is an autoimmune disease that is genetically inherited. It causes mood and body changes when the immune system "mistakenly attacks" the thyroid gland, causing overproduction of the thyroid hormones.

From Dr. Eva's Files

Elsa had recently given birth to her second child when she began to experience heart palpitations. She didn't think much about them until they began to appear more frequently. She went to a cardiologist who put her on heart medication. Unfortunately, the medication caused her blood pressure to drop so low that she had trouble getting out of bed in the morning and actually collapsed one afternoon with her child in her arms. With two young children to take care of, Elsa realized that the blood-pressure medication wasn't the best solution for her.

Elsa began to notice other symptoms as well. Although her husband had always described her as being "a little jumpy," she was now anxious all the time. She suffered from insomnia and unprovoked irritability. She went to see two other cardiologists because her palpitations were getting worse, but nothing seemed to help.

Her thyroid function was tested, but her results always came back within the normal range. Then one day, she went to see a nutritionist. After describing her symptoms, the nutritionist asked Elsa if she'd ever had a thyroid test. When told that her results were always normal, the nutritionist gave Elsa my number and said I might be able to help. After hearing Elsa's story, I decided to give her a series of thyroid tests during the week that we waited for her old medical records to arrive at my office. Sure enough, her first test result was "off the charts," and I suspected she had Graves' disease. A few more tests validated this diagnosis, and I soon had Elsa on the proper treatment plan. Within weeks she reported to me that she was feeling much better, was able to sleep through the night, and had not had any more heart palpitations. What she found interesting was that once we had gotten a hold of her prior doctor's medical records, there was no mention of thyroid labs ever being done. In retrospect, Elsa assumed that the doctor did thyroid labs because he said his lab testing was complete and that all was normal. My advice? When it comes to your doctor (even if that doctor is me), never assume.

People who have hyperthyroidism are often confused when they hear the diagnosis. My patients tell me, "I thought if I had hyperthyroidism, I'd be full of energy and losing weight and able to multitask like crazy! How come I'm so tired all the time?" Although this line of thinking is correct in most situations, the answer in other situations is that the overactive thyroid is burning out your body. It's negatively affecting other organs (such as the adrenal gland). It's like an engine that is constantly revving at a very high speed and going nowhere. Eventually, the parts will burn out and the engine will stop going (which seems to be what happened in Oprah's case).

Hyperthyroidism is treated by medication to calm the thyroid down, using drugs such as propylthiouracil (PTU) or Tapazole. You may need to have treatments with radioactive iodine, or with surgery to remove the thyroid gland. Some people need combinations of more than one treatment form. The condition can go into remission for many years. Relapses are uncommon but do occur.

Another type of hyperthyroidism is subacute thyroiditis, which involves swelling (inflammation) of the thyroid gland and is thought to be produced by a virus that usually follows an infection of the upper respiratory tract. It is often treated with anti-inflammatory drugs such as aspirin or ibuprofen to decrease both the production and the release of thyroid hormone. A beta-blocker (usually given for heart disease or hypertension or even tremors or anxiety) is also given to slow down the heart rate and make the patient more comfortable until the situation spontaneously resolves itself. This disease usually lasts for only a few months and heals itself naturally, but if left untreated, it can be life threatening.

TESTING YOUR THYROID

The good news is that there is a simple blood test that can measure thyroid function to determine whether or not your hormone production is normal (the "gold standard" is to test one of many thyroid functions, which is the production of thyroid stimulating hormone). The bad news is that if you get five doctors in a room, you'll get five different opinions on what is "normal" and what is not. In my practice, I don't rely on blood tests alone because over the years I have found that what is normal for one person, and even normal for the population at large, may be abnormal for someone else. I use other tests as well (such as one that tests for particular antibodies) and palpation (examining with my hands) of the thyroid to determine its size, shape, firmness, or location. Internists may do this as well, but since they do not palpate the gland as frequently as endocrinologists do, they may miss the diagnosis. Some doctors may recommend an ultrasound of the thyroid as well.

Here's where the tricky part comes in. As of 2010, at most laboratories in the United States, the official normal reference range for the thyroid-stimulating hormone blood test runs from approximately .5 to 5.0 (measured in micrograms per deciliter). Reference range is what determines—for the vast majority of physicians who rely almost exclusively on blood tests—whether or not thyroid disease is even diagnosed at all, much less treated, and when diagnosed, how it is treated. In January of 2003, the American Association of Clinical Endocrinologists recommended that doctors "consider treatment for patients who test outside the boundaries of a narrower margin based on a target TSH level of 0.3 to 3.0." Even though many years have passed since the new range was established, some doctors use it and some don't. The issue that it raises is this: One study found that when using a TSH upper-normal range of 5.0, approximately 5 percent of the population is hypothyroid. However, if you use 3.0 as the top of the normal range, approximately 20 percent of the population would be hypothyroid. That means that millions of patients with hypothyroidism are being undiagnosed and untreated.

Let's take my patient MaryAnn, for instance. When she was in her early 40s, she went to her doctor because she was feeling tired all the time and was having mood swings as well as irregular periods. The doctor suggested she have her thyroid tested, although he didn't really think that was the problem. MaryAnn's test results come back, and her TSH level was 4. According to the old standards, she was well within the normal reference range. So the doctor told MaryAnn she was fine and probably just needed a good rest. Ten years later, still living with fatigue, MaryAnn came to see me. Her symptoms had ramped up to a much higher level so that they now interfered with her daily life routine. I retested her thyroid; her TSH level had gone up to 5.0, and we agreed that she should begin treatment for hypothyroidism. Shortly thereafter, a new MaryAnn (or rather the one she used to know and love) returned. If MaryAnn's original doctor had gone by the new criteria, she would have been treated 10 years ago and had a much better quality of life. Instead, she had lived with symptoms for a decade, believing they were just part of the aging process.

There are now more effective blood tests that provide a complete picture of how well the thyroid produces T_4, how well the body converts T_4 into T_3, how much of the active form T_3 is created, and whether there are significant antithyroid antibodies present. A complete panel would also include levels of free (unbound) T_3 and T_4. You might want to suggest to your doctor that she use the free T_3 and T_4, as the "regular" T_3 and T_4 totals may not be as accurate.

One of the problems with thyroid testing is that the thyroid is typically not on the list of things that are regularly checked in a standard or even a more comprehensive blood test panel. Just like the guidelines we have established for testing for colon cancer, for instance, beginning at age 50 and not before, it's not until you reach the age of 65 that your doctor will routinely request thyroid testing. As we have said in other chapters, when you complain to your doctor about putting on weight, losing a little hair, fatigue, and lack of libido—most of the time you get the same response: "Well, you are getting older. It's to be expected." If you are suffering from any of these symptoms and your doctor doesn't suggest testing, bring it up yourself. Most doctors, even though they may be skeptical, will order the testing if you insist.

I Keep Forgetting What You Said About Thyroids . . .

Here is a frightening thought: many doctors have diagnosed patients with dementia and Alzheimer's disease, when in reality what they had was a thyroid disorder. A 2008 study published in the *Archives of Internal Medicine* found that older women who had levels of TSH that were either too high or too low had more than twice the risk of Alzheimer's disease than those with more moderate levels (the same was not true of men). This is another reason that testing your thyroid should become part of your standard medical routine as you get older!

Your Numbers, Your Doctor, and You

Here's an important point to remember if do get tested and your numbers are not "normal." Hypothyroidism has a huge range, from very mild to quite severe. Not only that, one person whose TSH tests result in a reading of 2.5 may feel perfectly fine, while another person with the same reading may be suffering a battery of symptoms. The numbers and the symptoms don't always correlate. Most of the time, taking thyroid medication will cure your symptoms, and you will feel better within a matter of days. By six weeks on the medication, you'll have a very good idea of how it's working. Unless you tell your doctor how you're feeling, he or she has nothing to go on but your test results. You need to share with your doctor if your symptoms are getting better (or worse), and you need to be consistently retested to see how your medication is working. Your numbers may go back to normal, but if you're still not feeling well, it's your responsibility to tell your doctor so that more tests can be taken or your medication can be tweaked.

It is possible, however, to go overboard with thyroid medication. Some of my patients have the "if some is good, more is better" attitude. However, too much thyroid medication can stress out the adrenal glands, which will then overproduce cortisol as well as dysregulate (impair) the ratio of cortisol, DHEA, epinephrine, and norepinephrine. This will leave you more fatigued than you were in the first place, because the rest of your body's systems will not be able to produce the energy needed to keep up with your now revved-up thyroid.

Iodine Deficiency and the Thyroid

Many years ago, I was traveling through the Himalayas, and I kept seeing people with large goiters on their necks. A goiter is an abnormal enlargement of the thyroid gland. In the Himalayas, I saw people with goiters that seemed bigger than their heads. They had to sleep almost upright so that they did not choke to death in the middle of the night. The sight of these people was one of the things that spurred my interest in endocrinology, and in the thyroid in particular.

The reason goiters were (and still are) so prevalent in these landlocked mountains is because of a lack of iodine in the diet. Since iodine is needed for the production of thyroid hormone, and the body does not make iodine, we have to get it through what we eat. It is commonly found in foods such as saltwater fish, seaweed, sea vegetables, shellfish, bread, cheese, and iodine-containing multivitamins. They do have bread and cheese in the Himalayas, but the cows eat the grass, which is iodine poor, and the bread is made from grains whose soil, once again, lacks iodine.

Iodized salt is now the main source of iodine in the American diet, but only about 20 percent of the salt America eats contains the micronutrient. Increasingly popular "designer" table salts, such as sea salts and Kosher salts, usually do not have much iodine. However, the majority of salt intake in the United States comes from processed foods, and food manufacturers almost always use noniodized salt in processed foods. Add to that the ubiquitous warnings against using too much salt because of our ever-pressing issues of hypertension, congestive heart disease, and other coronary artery diseases, and iodine deficiency becomes a real threat for some people in the United States. Whereas, just a few years ago iodine was mandated by the FDA to be included in salts (and was for decades), now most medical advice states that, due to the large variety of food sources available from all over the world, iodine in salt is no longer necessary in the United States and other Western countries. Iodization of salt is now voluntary in America. It appears that iodine intake has declined by 50 percent in North America in the past 30 to 40 years and the anticipated rate of future hypothyroid cases has risen dramatically.

Before the 1920s, iodine deficiency was common in the Great Lakes, Appalachian, and Northwestern regions of the United States and Canada; however, the introduction of iodized salt has virtually eliminated the problem in those areas. Iodine deficiency is more common in remote inland and mountainous regions of the world where food is grown in soil poor in iodine (e.g., areas like Bhutan, Tibet, and the Himalayas). Iodine deficiency can lead to goiter, hypothyroidism, and even to mental retardation in infants and children (the term "cretin" comes from the fetus not getting enough iodine while in the mother's womb).

Worldwide, the number one cause of hypothyroidism is iodine deficiency, which remains a public-health problem in 47 countries, and about 2.2 billion people (38 percent of the world's population) live in areas with iodine deficiency. An article in *The Lancet* in 2008 stated that, "According to WHO, in 2007, nearly 2 billion individuals had insufficient iodine intake, a third being of school age. . . . Thus iodine deficiency, as the single greatest preventable cause of mental retardation, is an important public-health problem."

There are many different types and brands of iodine supplementation available over the counter. It's important, however, that you get guidance from your doctor or health professional before taking any iodine supplementation. If you take too much, you can develop hyperthyroidism. You should never decide on your own how much iodine to take because you think it would increase your thyroid production. You might just do yourself more harm than good.

Your Thyroid and Your Baby

As every mother knows, there are a thousand and one things to worry about when you're pregnant. Well, here's another one: your thyroid and iodine deficiency. During pregnancy, thyroid hormone production increases by 50 percent, which means the body requires a greater intake of iodine to maintain thyroid function and thyroid hormone production.

In 2007, the World Health Organization (WHO), the United Nations Children's Fund (UNICEF), and the International Council for the Control of Iodine Deficiency Disorders (ICCIDD) issued a publication called "Assessment of iodine deficiency disorders and monitoring their elimination," in which they outlined the result of iodine deficiency in pregnancy and lactation:

❖ Spontaneous abortion

❖ Stillbirth

❖ Congenital anomalies

❖ Perinatal mortality

❖ Endemic cretinism

❖ Impaired mental function

❖ Delayed physical development

The 2007 publication also states: "On a worldwide basis, iodine deficiency is the single most important preventable cause of brain damage. People living in areas affected by severe iodine deficiency may have an intelligence quotient (IQ) of up to 13.5 points below that of those from comparable communities in areas where there is no iodine deficiency."

Thyroid problems can continue to haunt a woman even after she gives birth. As much as 10 percent of all postpartum emotional and physical complaints are caused by thyroid imbalances. This type of hypothyroidism usually lasts for several months and then rights itself. However, in some cases it can require long-term treatment.

In 2006, the American Thyroid Association published guidelines recommending that all pregnant and breastfeeding women take prenatal vitamins containing iodine, but few women are aware of the recommendation. Women who have already been diagnosed as hypothyroid and are on thyroid medication typically need to increase their thyroid supplementation by 50 percent during pregnancy. Immediately after giving birth, they usually go back to their original dosage.

In the U.S., the recommended daily allowance (RDA) for iodine for adults is 150 mcg/day, 220 mcg/day for pregnant women, and 290 mcg/day for lactating women. Based on those guidelines, many prenatal vitamins do not have sufficient iodine for the average woman. Even mild iodine deficiency during pregnancy may be associated with lower intelligence in children, which is why I monitor my pregnant hypothyroid patients every two months to check on their thyroid and levels, and that's why, if you are pregnant, you should be sure to ask your doctor to test your thyroid levels and to be sure that you are getting enough iodine to keep your baby healthy.

Thyroid Treatments

One of the first thyroid treatments that was commercially available was Armour Thyroid, which was a natural product made of desiccated pig and cow thyroid glands put into pill form. It is still available today. It contains both T_3 and T_4 hormones. It fell out of favor over the years because quality control of this medication was difficult. In recent years, however, production has become much more stable, and it is back in use again. Your doctor may prescribe Armour Thyroid if you have had problems with a synthetic therapy, or if you or your doctor prefer natural products.

Armour Thyroid should be prescribed by a physician. Some health-food and natural-food stores sell glandular product supplements; however, I do not recommend using them as they are frequently not regulated by the Food and Drug Administration, and their potency and purity are usually not guaranteed.

The most commonly prescribed synthetic drug for hypothyroidism is called levothyroxine, known under the brand names Synthroid, Levothroid, Levoxyl, and Unithroid. A more recent addition is a drug called Tirosint, which is made in Switzerland and distributed in the United States. It has fewer additives and preservatives than the other synthetic medications, so it may be a good choice for you if you find you're allergic to any of the other brands.

Another popular drug is called Cytomel, which contains only T_3. Synthroid contains only T_4, which must be converted to T_3 by the body. Some people respond better to T_3 preparations because they have trouble converting T_4 into T_3; those people fare better with either a combination of T_3/T_4 or T_3 alone.

The mineral selenium decreases the antibodies that form in Hashimoto's thyroiditis, thereby decreasing the inflammation, which is why I recommend selenium to everyone who has hypothyroidism. It is also useful as a messenger in the brain helping with the communication between the thyroid and the adrenal gland.

How to Take Thyroid Medication

Although thyroid problems are usually easily treated with medication, it can be tricky to take because of how thyroid hormones react with other substances. Tell your doctor about all the prescription and over-the-counter medications you use because there are many other medicines that can affect thyroid medications. This includes vitamins, minerals, and herbal products. There are also some substances that block the absorption of thyroid medications (e.g., soy, calcium, iron, some mood-altering prescription medications), which is why some patients don't see the results they'd like.

❖ Do not take thyroid medication within two hours of eating as food may delay or reduce its absorption.

❖ Do not take estrogen, birth-control pills, or hormone-replacement therapy in the pill form at the same time you're taking thyroid medication (you can take them in the same day, just not at the same time of the day). Any form of oral estrogen may be a problem if taken at the same time as thyroid medication because both estrogen and thyroid hormone share the same binding globulin (a protein to which thyroid hormone binds in the blood and from which it is released into tissue cells) in the liver. If you take them both at the same time, you're not absorbing as much of either one. This does not apply if you are taking other forms of birth control, such as the patch or the NuvaRing; transdermal (through the skin) hormone replacement; or sublingual (dissolving directly into the bloodstream from drops or lozenges in the mouth) hormone replacement. That's another reason why I treat my menopausal women who have hypothyroidism with a hormone *cream* instead of the standard oral prescription pill.

❖ Calcium also prevents absorption of thyroid medication, so they should not be taken at the same time. If you are on thyroid replacement medication, you must be on a higher dosage of daily calcium replacement than if you are not on thyroid medication. No matter what your age, you should have a total of 1,500 mg of calcium daily. Unfortunately, most calcium brands can only be absorbed at 500 mg at one dosage. So even if your tablet says 800 mg, you may still be absorbing only 500 mg. This means that you have to supplement yourself at three distinct times a day—which becomes difficult when you also have to stay clear of thyroid medication at the same time. So don't beat yourself up trying to accomplish this goal. Do the best you can and make sure you have your bone density monitored routinely.

❖ Iron, whether alone, or as part of a multivitamin or prenatal vitamin supplement, interferes with thyroid hormone absorption. You should not take your iron supplements or your vitamins with iron at the same time as your thyroid hormone. You should allow at least two hours (four being the optimal time frame) between taking them.

YOUR THYROID AND MENOPAUSE

Although it is very rarely mentioned, your thyroid and your reproductive cycle are closely related. Thyroid problems can cause irregularities in the menstrual cycle and even infertility in extreme cases. As you get older, these problems can become exacerbated. In fact, untreated hypothyroidism can cause a woman to be in an artificial premature perimenapause or even throw her into menopause.

It's important to remember that the thyroid is part of the overall endocrine system, and when any of this system's hormones get out of balance, all of the parts suffer. So when you go through times where hormonal imbalance is more than likely—such as pregnancy, perimenopause, and menopause—your thyroid is also more than likely to get out of whack.

That is why women over 50 should be tested for thyroid problems every few years (earlier if you have a family history) and women over 65 should be tested annually. Any woman of any age should be tested at any time and as frequently as needed if she has symptoms of hypothyroidism. Your doctor will then be able to determine whether you need thyroid hormone medication, and/ or iodine or other supplementation.

In dealing with thyroid problems, it's important to find a doctor who will listen to your symptoms and be open to the newest research, the latest reference range recommendations, inclusive testing, and who understands that each patient will react differently to various treatments. You may need to see an endocrinologist to get the results you need and deserve.

It makes me frustrated to know that there are so many women who suffer unnecessarily for so many years. I hear it over and over again, how finally being diagnosed and treated for thyroid problems has changed women's lives. They have accepted their "lot in life" for so long that they have almost forgotten what it's like to have energy and focus and fun in their lives. I'm here to tell you, don't just accept it. Get tested. Check your results. Ask for a copy of your labs. See a specialist. Don't settle—if you don't agree with your doctor, go somewhere else. You know your body better than anyone else. Listen to it, and get your life and your health back in your hands.

THE CHECK YOUR THYROID
jump-start tips

1. **Taking Matters into Your Own Hands—or Armpits.** If you suspect you're having thyroid problems and you want to check yourself out at home, there is a simple test you can do called the basal temperature test. Here are the steps:

   - Get a basal thermometer (the kind you can use under your tongue). Leave it overnight on your bedside table.

   - First thing in the morning, before you get out of bed, tuck the thermometer under your armpit and lay completely still for 10 minutes. Set a timer before you begin so that you don't have to move around to look at the clock.

   - Record your temperature for three to five days. If your temperature is consistently below 97.8°F, you may have a thyroid problem, and you should have yourself evaluated by a health professional.

2. **Iodine: The Home Test.** There is a simple and inexpensive way you can test yourself for iodine deficiency:

  ♦ Dip a cotton ball into USP Tincture of Iodine. (Use the orange-tinted kind, not the clear version. You can get iodine at the drugstore. If you can't find it, ask the pharmacist.)

  ♦ Paint a 2- to 3-inch circle of iodine on your abdomen, the inner part of your thigh, or your upper arm.

  ♦ You will see a yellow-orange stain on your skin. If the stain takes four to six hours to disappear, your iodine level is fine. If it disappears within one to three hours, you may be iodine deficient. If that is the case, the next step is to ask your health-care provider for the more accurate, 24-hour iodine/iodide loading test.

3. **Try Yoga.** There are several alternative treatments that, used in conjunction with doctor-recommended medications, are helpful to people with thyroid problems. Many people find that yoga can stimulate the thyroid gland to work at its peak efficiency. One specific pose that is thought to be of great benefit to the thyroid is known as a shoulder stand, or sarvangasan. To perform a yoga shoulder stand, lie flat on your back, keep your legs together, and raise your legs until they are at a right angle to your shoulders/neck, perpendicular to the floor. Tuck your chin into your chest, and rest the weight of your body on your shoulders and elbows, using your arms to support your hips. Try to practice until you can do a shoulder stand for a full two minutes.

4. **Try acupuncture.** As mentioned earlier, acupuncture has a wide host of benefits. The World Health Organization lists over 40 diseases that acupuncture can treat effectively, and thyroid is on the list. Acupuncture is often used to help stimulate the

immune system, which makes it a good choice for treating Hashimoto's thyroiditis, an autoimmune disorder. Acupuncture can also be useful for treating symptoms of hypothyroid, even if the condition itself is not addressed in the treatment. For instance, acupuncture is noted for increasing energy and decreasing stress, both of which are helpful for people with hypothyroidism. It can also help with some of the menstrual irregularities that sometimes come with hypothyroidism. Although this may be your preferential treatment, you should still consult with your medical doctor routinely to make sure that your hormones are responding appropriately. Remember, thyroid disease is not just about fatigue, it can ultimately affect your morbidity as well as your mortality. Take control, but do it with the assistance of an expert.

Speaking of menstrual irregularities . . . the next chapter is all about how your hormones affect your cycles—your monthly cycle as well as your cycle of life. Whether you're worried about getting your period or not getting your period, Chapter 8 will give you the basics and maybe help you feel better and feel better about yourself no matter what cycle you're in.

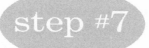

step #7

Prepare Yourself for That Time of the Month (Or That Time of Your Life)

Most women remember the day they got their first period. It's a rite of passage: the physical evidence that they are transitioning from girls to women. In fact, there are still many countries where, once a girl gets her period, she's likely to be wed or sold off. Her education may be stopped, or she may be pulled out of school and put to work, either in the home or out in the world. It is something to be feared. Even in the 21st century, many women around the globe have primitive notions of "that time of the month." A study of young women in Pakistan in 2010 found that almost 13 percent of the participants perceived menstruation as a disease and a curse from God. In Taiwan, a 2009 study showed that there was a significant negative correlation between menstrual attitudes and menstrual distress. In other words, the young women who thought the worst about getting their periods felt the worst when they actually got their periods.

Although I remember the day very well, I can't remember exactly how old I was when I got my first period. I know I was a late bloomer. And I know it was an emotional time for me. I remember being upset because it meant I was no longer a young child. There was a sense of security in being a little girl that I didn't want to lose. I thought my relationship with my parents would change, and I liked things just the way they were.

A good friend of mine recalls having to wear what she remembers as a huge pad because she didn't know how to deal with her bleeding in any other way. She went to school one day and forgot her brick-sized pad and had "an accident." She was incredibly embarrassed and afraid that all the boys would know, so she ran out of school, rode her bike home (a mile away), changed her clothes, and rode back to school. Instead of embracing the power of being a woman, she resented it. She was humiliated, and she isolated herself at "that time of the month" so that this horrific episode of her life would never be repeated. A lot of baggage for a 13-year-old girl. Some mothers still tell their daughters not to wear a tampon because they claim that it will make them lose their virginity. It is possible, although unlikely, that inserting a tampon may tear the hymen, but that does not affect virginity. Virginity is related to sexual intercourse; it has nothing to do with the use of tampons. Many young girls, even in the United States in the 21st century, are still wearing napkins instead of tampons, which really limits their participation in sports and their overall lifestyle.

THE CYCLE BEGINS

It doesn't matter how old you are or where you are in the world, the onset of menstruation—the beginning of the cycle of womanhood—brings changes, both physical and emotional, to your life. These changes are all due to hormones.

If you haven't figured this out from the previous chapters of this book, I'll lay it out for you straight and simple: a woman's life is all about hormones (a man's too, but their hormones are more like an on/off switch, whereas a woman's hormones are more like the dashboard of a fighter jet, tons of switches everywhere). We live a life of delicate balance. When one hormone is active, another one is less active. Many of our hormones naturally cycle so that at certain times of the day or the month, they course through our bodies at higher or lower levels, depending on what the body needs at that particular moment. It's a well-oiled machine.

Except when it's not.

Because our hormones function in such tenuous equilibrium, it's not uncommon for one hormone or another to fluctuate to the point of a dangerous imbalance. When that happens, it can disrupt our daily lives. Hormone balance is affected by every single thing we do. It can be thrown off by what you eat or what you don't eat, by how much you exercise or how sedentary you are, or by how much stress there is in your life and how well you handle it. Although at first glance that may not seem like good news, it is. Because these are things you can change and control. You can adjust your diet. You can get more exercise. You can change your attitude toward things that worry you or modify your behavior so that you can better cope with life's stressors. And in some cases, you can use hormone supplementation, whether prescription or herbal, to help bring your body back into balance.

It's important to remember that there are many different hormones at work in our bodies at the same time. We are much more than just our reproductive glands; our bodies produce nearly 100 different types of hormones. There isn't one magic hormone (or one magic food, supplement, medication, or vitamin) that will keep us youthful and energized or protect us from all the ways we sabotage ourselves. Similarly, there is no one lifestyle factor that will cure us of all our ills—it is the combination of factors, including diet, exercise, and personal habits, that makes for a balanced lifestyle and a balanced endocrine system.

Hormones originate from various glands throughout the body. As we learned in Chapter 1, they circulate through your bloodstream and come in contact with all your cells; however, only certain target cells react because they have receptors for that particular hormone. If the receptors become overly sensitive, cells can become overloaded with a particular hormone and the reaction of the cell can become abnormally intense. Conversely, if the receptors become desensitized, cells will not get their customary hormonal load and will not react as strongly as they should. Both of these situations can cause a whole host of problems.

There have been huge volumes written on the subjects of PMS, perimenopause, and menopause. This book would be incomplete without touching on these subjects, but by no means do I suggest that this is a complete analysis (so watch out for the next book!).

THE SEX HORMONES

In this chapter, we are revisiting several of the body's hormones that are involved in a woman's reproductive cycles. These hormones are important not just for having babies, but for much of the energy production and the overall health (physical and mental) of a woman's life.

Estrogen

Although most women think of *estrogen* as the most important reproductive hormone, the term actually applies to many different distinct compounds. Three of the most important ones are estradiol, estriol, and estrone.

❖ Estradiol is the primary sex hormone of childbearing women; it is responsible for female characteristics and sexual functioning. Estradiol is also important to women's bone health. An imbalance of estradiol contributes to many gynecologic problems such as endometriosis and fibroids and even female cancers.

❖ Estriol is only produced in significant amounts during pregnancy as it is made by the placenta. Levels of estriol in nonpregnant women do not change much after menopause. Estrone and estradiol stimulate the cell growth necessary for reproduction. However, when found in too high a level they can be carcinogenic (cancer-causing). Estriol, on the other hand, has been found to protect the body from the harmful effects of estrone and estradiol, and estriol has been shown to be anticarcinogenic. Estriol has been used in cream form for vaginal dryness and urinary tract problems in menopausal women in Europe for 30 years, and its safety and effectiveness are well established.

❖ Estrone is widespread throughout the body. It is the only one of the estrogens that's present in any significant amount in women after menopause. This form of estrogen seems to work best for diminishing hot flashes, but it is also the one most associated with a risk for breast cancer. If you are choosing a hormone-replacement therapy, my usual recommendation is a combination of estriol and estradiol, without estrone.

If you want to think about a source of power, you've got to think about estrogen. Almost all tissues in the body have estrogen receptors. However, hormone levels ebb and flow throughout the day. Estrogen is secreted in short bursts, which means that levels vary from hour to hour and even minute to minute. Hormone levels are different during the night than in the day and from one stage of the menstrual cycle to another.

Estrogen levels start to rise in girls at about the age of 8, well before their first period, which normally begins at around age 11 or 12. That's also when girls begin to develop breasts and grow pubic hair and hair under their arms. Estrogen may begin to drop when women are in their early-to-mid-30s, decline more rapidly as women reach their 40s, and reach nearly zero when they are in their 50s. Low estrogen levels can affect your physical energy, leaving you fatigued for no apparent reason. You may feel that you cannot concentrate enough to finish any task or that you need to take an afternoon nap. By the time you're in your 50s and have hit menopause, you may have difficulty getting to sleep, wake up several times during the night, and still feel tired in the morning. For many women "the light is on but nobody's home."

Low estrogen levels also decrease the body's ability to create new bone cells, which puts a woman at an increased risk of developing osteoporosis. Estrogen is also cardioprotective, meaning that estrogen protects women from heart disease. It's the reason women outlive men in general. It saves us from cardiac disease and stroke. When estrogen levels fall, the risk of these diseases rises.

Progesterone

Progesterone is secreted by the corpus luteum (a mass of cells that forms on the ovary at the place where an egg is released) after ovulation. Progesterone is meant to prepare the uterus for pregnancy, among other things. If pregnancy occurs, progesterone production is eventually provided by the placenta. If pregnancy doesn't occur, the corpus luteum disintegrates and you begin menstruation within 12 to 16 days.

Progesterone also serves several other important functions in the body. It helps regulate the thyroid gland, enhances the immune system, reduces swelling and inflammation, and keeps blood-clotting levels at normal values. Progesterone helps produce collagen and helps stabilize nerve functions.

Normally, estrogen and progesterone levels both rise starting at the time of ovulation until just before menstruation. If there is a low level of progesterone, that means there will be a higher estrogen to progesterone ratio, and that can cause a variety of symptoms, including fibroid and tumor development, increases in cholesterol levels, low blood-sugar levels, fluid retention, and fatigue.

As you get older, your levels of both progesterone and estrogen begin to decline. This gradually leads to menopause.

Testosterone

Testosterone, the "male" sex hormone, is also produced in smaller amounts in women's bodies, mostly by the ovaries and adrenal glands. Men produce about 20 times as much testosterone per day as women do. As we know, testosterone is not just for sex—it plays an important role in a woman's health and well-being, not to mention her energy production. As we age, most women experience a decrease in testosterone, which reduces our sexual libido, increases the risk of depression, contributes to bone loss, causes muscle weakness, and results in a general loss of vital energy.

HIJACKED BY HORMONES: PMS

Before you get your period, do you:

❖ Experience feelings of anxiety and irritability characteristic of mood swings?

❖ Often feel sad or lethargic?

❖ Find that your breasts feel tender?

❖ Experience bloating?

❖ Get headaches or uterine pain?

❖ Crave sweets or salty foods?

If you answered "yes" to two or more of these questions, you know all about irritability and overreaction to small annoyances, feeling sad before your period, the weird food cravings, and the bloating and the cramps. These are all the cyclical, physical, and emotional symptoms associated with premenstrual syndrome (PMS), which is caused by hormonal imbalance. According to a study in the *Archives of Internal Medicine,* as many as 90 percent of women experience some symptoms before their period. That's a huge number of women. Of this group an estimated 5 to 12 percent will experience severe, incapacitating PMS. Approximately 10 percent of women will experience no symptoms at all.

No two women experience menstruation in the same way, and no two women's cycles are identical. A lot depends on a woman's genetics, her diet, her lifestyle, and her stress levels. However, the medical explanation of how the body functions before, during, and after menstruation remains the same for all women. Here is a short refresher course on what happens during that time of the month and when PMS occurs:

❖ The average age for the first period is about 12 ½ years old. The average age for the last period is about 51 years old.

❖ The menstrual cycle is defined as beginning on the first day of a woman's period and ending on the last day before her next period.

❖ There are two phases to each menstrual cycle: the follicular phase and the luteal phase.

❖ The follicular phase begins on the day your period starts and lasts for about 14 days. When this phase begins, estrogen and progesterone are at their lowest levels. Estrogen rises in this first half of the cycle and peaks at ovulation. During this phase, there is a higher ratio of estrogen to progesterone. This is often a time of high energy.

❖ The luteal phase begins on day 14, after ovulation occurs, and continues until day 1 of your next period. Estrogen falls in this second half of the cycle as progesterone rises and prepares the lining of the uterus for the implantation of a fertilized egg, should conception occur. During this phase, there is a higher ratio of progesterone to estrogen, and this is usually when PMS begins. If pregnancy does not occur, the lining of the uterus begins to shed, which leads to menstruation.

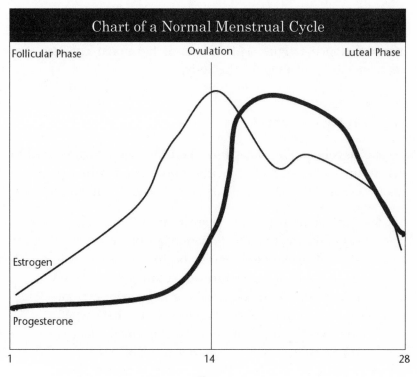

Like many other things in life, most women assume PMS is a natural part of life, and they deal with it, take painkillers, or call in sick to work or school. Some women practically shut down their lives for a week, but they don't really seek out how to conquer their PMS, which can range from headaches to cramping to feeling like a pithed frog, pinned down and alive but not able to move. And utterly exhausted. Typically, PMS occurs right before or at the onset of menstruation, but you can have it during ovulation as well. Some women get it at ovulation *and* right before their menstrual cycle; their whole lives seem to revolve around PMS.

If you talk to any woman about energy (or lack of it), the subject of "that time of the month" inevitably arises. For many women, the days just before they get their period are marked by a variety of symptoms, including, very often, a profound sense of lethargy. PMS has as many as 150 different symptoms. For most women, the most disturbing symptoms seem to be irritability, mood swings, depression, water retention, and breast tenderness, as well as the aforementioned fatigue. This is due to hormonal changes that cause metabolic changes in the body.

Why Do We Get PMS?

We've come a long way since the time when doctors used to debate the reality of PMS, but the short answer is that there are many reasons why PMS occurs. There are several different theories:

❖ **Decline in progesterone levels.** PMS symptoms occur during the luteal phase of a woman's cycle, which is when progesterone begins to rise (right after ovulation) and then starts to plummet about seven days later. When you are about to get your period, your progesterone levels rapidly drop. That's what causes problems. Hormone levels normally fluctuate. If progesterone levels were measured on a scale of 1 to 10, for example, they could drop from a level of 10 to a 9.9 to a 9.8 to a 9.7 and your body would be able to adjust to the changing levels with almost no difficulty. When you're about to get your period, however, levels drop dramatically from a 10 to a 5 and perhaps even to a 1. It's that rapid change that stimulates your symptoms. And some women drop faster and lower than others, which is why their symptoms may be worse than other women's.

❖ **Decrease in neurotransmitters serotonin and GABA activity.** Serotonin is responsible for our positive emotional well-being, while GABA helps keeps us calm. Reduced levels of estrogen during the luteal phase may be linked to a drop in serotonin. Lower serotonin levels are associated with irritability, anger, and carbohydrate cravings, all of which are symptoms of PMS. It also appears that GABA receptors are less sensitive than normal, which would explain the increased sense of anxiety.

❖ **Changes in levels of norepinephrine and epinephrine.** These neurotransmitters are involved in the body's stress response. Estrogen may affect the levels of these neurotransmitters, which can influence blood pressure and heart rate as well as mood.

Other possible causes of PMS includeinclude:

❖ Hypoglycemia (low blood sugar)

❖ Mercury toxicity

❖ Hypothyroidism

❖ Candida overgrowth (a fungus)

❖ Food allergies/sensitivities

❖ Vitamin B$_6$, calcium, or magnesium deficiencies

❖ Inadequate protein intake—liver enzymes that convert female hormones depend on protein

❖ Poor liver function—the liver metabolizes one form of estrogen into other forms of estrogen

❖ Poor adrenal-gland function

No one knows for sure what causes PMS. Some people attribute particular symptoms to increased levels of estrogen and/or progesterone; other people say the same symptom is due to decreased levels of these hormones. Studies routinely produce conflicting results. I believe that the key to eliminating or greatly reducing PMS symptoms lies in the balance between these two hormones during the menstrual cycle.

PMS and the Fatigue Factor

Although the specific symptoms of PMS vary from woman to woman, fatigue is one of the top three complaints women have—the other two being irritability (many of my patients use the term *raving bitch*) and bloating. As you can see from the chart on page 217, estrogen levels fluctuate quite a bit in both phases of the menstrual cycle. The drop in estrogen affects the adrenal gland (most estrogen is produced in the ovaries; however, the adrenal glands do produce a small amount of the hormone) as well as transmission of neuropeptides, small proteinlike molecules used by neurons to communicate with each other—all of which exhausts your body's energy. When estrogen levels drop, they have a negative effect on the stress hormone cortisol. The combination of low estrogen and the dysfunctional surge of cortisol can cause a state of chronic deep exhaustion.

PMS-related fatigue has also been associated with magnesium deficiency. Estrogen enhances the utilization of magnesium. However, if estrogen levels are low, which is often the case during PMS, magnesium may not be utilized properly by the body. Studies have shown that there are significantly lower concentrations of magnesium in women who have PMS than that of control groups. High-magnesium foods help relax the muscles in turn helping with the effects of PMS cramps. Such foods include:

❖ Pumpkin, sesame, and sunflower seeds

❖ Greens such as spinach, broccoli, okra, Swiss chard, and artichokes

❖ Halibut and tuna

❖ Almonds, Brazil nuts, and pine nuts

❖ Black and navy beans

The good news is that there are a number of things you can do about PMS. PMS fatigue is part of the body's normal response to the changes that occur during your monthly cycle. It's a signal that changes are happening inside your body. Like any other signal your body may give you, you have the opportunity to listen to it and respond appropriately. Here are some tips for dealing with PMS and the fatigue that my accompany it:

❖ **Diet:** If you suffer from any of the symptoms of PMS, not just fatigue, you can help decrease their effects by what and when you eat. The most important thing you want to do for PMS is to keep your hormones on an even keel as much as possible. That means eating every three to four hours and following the Fatigue Solution philosophy of having a protein at every meal as well as complex carbohydrates and unsaturated fats. Also, remember to use these helpful hints:

- **Eat a variety of foods.** It's important to eat a variety of foods every day, including iron-rich foods, such as red meat, egg yolks, spinach, broccoli, leafy greens, prunes, raisins, beans, beets, squash, and yams. If you eat iron-rich foods along with foods that provide plenty of vitamin C, your body can better absorb the iron.

- **Fill up on fruits and veggies.** Eating more fruits and vegetables will help increase essential mineral and vitamin intake.

- **Up your fiber.** Increasing fiber intake will help reduce the absorption rate of glucose into the bloodstream to smooth out blood-sugar highs and lows.

- **Eat more complex carbs.** Increasing the amount of complex carbohydrates (e.g., vegetables and whole grains) in your diet can help increase levels of serotonin. Low serotonin levels have been linked to PMS-related depression and mood swings.

- **Ditch the salt.** Decreasing salt will help prevent bloating and fluid retention. This will also help lower high blood pressure. Some of my patients use diuretics (drugs that tend to increase the flow of urine, which causes the body to get rid of excess water) to decrease bloating, which they take right before their period and for the first few days after flow begins. Using a low-dose infrequent diuretic is relatively safe, but these are prescription drugs that can be overused, so always consult with your physician about whether or not it's right for you.

◆ **Eat naturally.** Reduce consumption of processed foods and refined sugar, which are rapidly converted into glucose and can cause intense fluctuations in blood sugar levels. Sugar makes processing estrogen more difficult for the body, and causes blood sugar to rise too quickly.

◆ **Say good-bye to caffeine.** Avoid caffeinated drinks, which can exacerbate sleep problems and the resultant fatigue. Caffeine can also cause dehydration and reduce iron absorption. Reducing caffeine can also help alleviate breast tenderness.

❖ **Exercise:** Exercise is often the last thing you feel like doing when you're dealing with PMS, but exercise increases serotonin and endorphins, which provide feelings of well-being. This could be the reason that women who exercise have fewer premenstrual symptoms. You may have to go lighter or easier but you still should try to get a moderate workout in every few days during your PMS and cycle. Here are some exercise tips for dealing with PMS:

◆ **Take a dip in the pool.** A low-resistance water workout can be just what you need to give your muscles a workout at the same time you increase your overall feelings of well-being.

◆ **Try yoga.** The stretching aspects of yoga can help to manage cramps, while the meditative properties can help you feel calmer and less irritable.

◆ **Experience Pilates.** Do your joints and muscles ache before you get your period? Pilates helps to elongate the body using gentle, nonaerobic movements, which can help relieve those aches and pains.

- **Kick out your frustrations.** While some women benefit most from gentle movements, others find that an all-out, sweat-producing, highly active session of kickboxing is exactly what they need to get over the feelings of anger and irritability that often accompany PMS.

- **Hire a personal trainer.** This may be the perfect time to have someone else there to motivate you and keep you going just when you're least likely to get up off the couch. Even if it's for one day a month (during the week before your period), knowing you have to be accountable to a trainer—not to mention the fact that you're paying him or her good money—will keep you from sabotaging yourself with too little exercise and too many fattening "treats."

Treating PMS with Hormones

In my practice, I often have young women who come to me complaining that they are not just tired when they get PMS, they are so exhausted they can't function at all for at least a week every month. For a patient who falls into this group, I recommend a salivary test that can help us define what is going on hormonally during her cycle (see Chapter 9 for more on this test). It will help us determine whether she has a progesterone problem or an estrogen problem, or issues with testosterone or DHEA as well as where in the cycle (what time of the month) these hormones need to be replaced. This approach can be handled by cycling bioidentical hormones (which are different compounds than the bioidenticals we talk about when we discuss menopausal hormone replacement, so don't get confused). Most often, when a woman complains of this kind of extreme symptom, her hormones are in dire need of being leveled out. In that case, the quickest, easiest and, at times, most effective treatment is usually to put her on birth-control pills to even out ovarian hormone fluctuations.

Some alternative medicine doctors don't like the idea of putting their patients on birth-control pills. There has been some negative press, but overall it is still the easiest, most economical, most benign way of dealing with PMS. There may be some ramifications of taking the pill, such as decreased libido, but we can deal with that (see Chapter 5). Otherwise, I don't think it's necessary for a woman to suffer with debilitating symptoms. I usually suggest lower-estrogen pills that have been shown in studies to have a significant impact on mood and physical symptoms or those that extend the length of cycles so that the women on them bleed every 12 weeks rather than every four. Birth-control pills, however, do not resolve any core imbalances that underlie these issues. That means that these pills provide temporary relief for extreme symptoms, but that you should be working on imbalance issues at the same time, through lifestyle changes, stress management, and exercise.

Alternative Therapies for PMS

A fairly new entry into the treatment for PMS is light therapy. Light therapy consists of exposure for up to an hour a day to high intensity light from a light box made specifically for that purpose. Light therapy users sit 12 to 24 inches away from the light source. PMS sufferers focus on light treatment in the luteal phase which precedes menstruation. Light therapy used in this way provides significant relief of PMS depression and reduces the symptoms of premenstrual tension.

Another thing to keep in mind is that because hormones have to travel through the liver to be broken down into their most effective forms, having a "clean" liver helps with PMS as well. Herbs that can help cleanse the liver include milk thistle (which may help the liver metabolize estrogen, thereby reducing the symptoms of PMS), dandelion, and burdock root.

THE NEXT PHASE: PERIMENOPAUSE

When a single friend of mine was in her mid-40s, she missed a period. She knew she wasn't pregnant, as she hadn't been dating for months. Then she had one hot flash. She became hysterical, sure that she was going through early menopause. She actually went to see four different doctors (including me). All of the doctors (including me) assured her that what she was experiencing was absolutely normal. She was not menopausal, but her body was starting its progression, and sometime within the next two to ten years, she would be entering the no-more-periods zone. But not quite yet.

My friend was in perimenopause, meaning she had begun the years leading up to menopause, during which levels of female hormones fluctuate more widely than normal from month to month as hormone production gradually decreases and periods become irregular. One concern that women have once they're in their 40s is that they think they're going into premature or early menopause because their cycle gets shorter and changes from 28 days to 21 days. They tell me that their period is lighter and/or shorter than it used to be, or that it's heavy one month and light the next and then heavy again. All these changes have to do with perimenopause.

The PerimenoQuiz

Have you:

- ❖ Missed your period during the last few cycles?
- ❖ Had several heavier or lighter periods than usual?
- ❖ Noticed that your skin is drier or oilier than usual?
- ❖ Woken up hot and sweaty in the middle of the night?
- ❖ Been less than enthusiastic about sex?
- ❖ Experienced any heart palpitations or flutters in the last six months?

❖ Been moodier, more irritable, or more depressed than usual?

❖ Felt exhausted no matter how much sleep you get?

If you answered "yes" to two or more of these questions, you may be experiencing perimenopause. Some women hardly even know they're in perimenopause. They may begin to skip periods, but otherwise have no symptoms. About 80 percent of women in their 40s begin skipping their period altogether. Interestingly enough, about 10 percent of women go from completely normal cycles to stopping menstruation altogether. But no one can tell you what to expect from your perimenopausal years—you just have to wait until you get there to know how you will react.

One patient in perimenopause told me, "I feel like digging a hole and climbing into it." Another said, "I feel like I'm living outside my head." And yet another patient stated that, although she was calm on the outside, her insides were jumping around. She was extremely anxious and depressed even though she had nothing to be unhappy about. She had a gorgeous, wealthy husband, she was a stay-at-home mom with fabulous kids and no mortgage to worry about, and she had housekeepers to cook and clean for her. Yet her insides were jumping around creating extreme anxiety. Hormones were wreaking havoc with all these women, each in their own way.

Think of these changing hormones as an opportunity to reevaluate your life. Understand that the changes you make during this period of time will help you with the changes you may need to make when you enter into menopause.

When you go through perimenopause, your cycle will change. The number of days between periods may become shorter; you may start having your period every three weeks instead of every four. The brain becomes less sensitive to estrogen; therefore, the follicle stimulating hormones have to work harder so that the amount of estrogen is maintained. The amount of estrogen remains the same, but the brain is working a lot harder to produce it. That's also one of the ways we can determine whether or not a woman is fertile, by looking at her follicle stimulating hormone (FSH) level. The higher it is, the less likely fertility can occur.

It's Not Your Age That Counts

I recently had 42-year-old woman in my office who was premenopausal. I also had a patient who was 49 years old, and she was suffering from PMS. I had a 38-year-old patient who had gone through menopause. The doctor she had been seeing listened to her symptoms and then told her, "You're too young to be menopausal." I can't emphasize strongly enough that every woman is different. There is no age-based definition that tells you when you are premenopausal or when you are going to stop having your period. A good doctor will listen to your symptoms and then suggest you have your hormones tested, which will tell you what's happening with your body. There is no such thing as "You're too young for this," or "You're too old for that." Your diagnosis really should be symptom specific, not age specific.

At the same time, your levels of progesterone start to decrease during perimenopause. But it's not just the fact that you're losing progesterone that causes symptoms; it's the fact that the ratio of other hormones to progesterone is increasing. So you may have the same amount of estrogen as you had before, but the ratio is now higher, causing estrogen dominance. Many times, women will seek out estrogen therapy or go to an herbalist who suggests soy products because they're interpreting perimenopause as an estrogen deficiency. What they end up doing, however, is aggravating an already bad situation. Remember, soy acts as an estrogen, so in a sense, by adding soy to your diet, you are adding more fuel to the fire.

Perimenopause is really about hormonal surges. One day your estrogen can be high, the next day it can be low. It's these surges that create mood swings and cause us to want to eat more and exercise less, which in turn shows up as "unexplained" weight gain.

These hormonal surges are also responsible for our emotions going wild. Your hormones are erratic, to say the least. In the past, your hormones may have stayed at a particular level for several days; now they may remain stationary for no more than a few hours at a time.

This can lead to extreme situations. Kimberly came to me recently for a second opinion. She was 43 years old, and wanted to get a total hysterectomy, meaning she voluntarily wanted to have both her uterus and ovaries removed. It seems that for the past five years, she had been losing abnormally large amounts of blood during her period and suffering from horrible mood swings and depression. She had tried several types of birth-control pills as well as an IUD, and nothing controlled her bleeding. Her ob-gyn told her that her moods were due to depression and prescribed her Prozac, which made her feel worse. It was the patient who suggested the total hysterectomy, and shockingly, her doctor had agreed!

She wanted the hysterectomy because she couldn't deal with the excessive bleeding. Not only did she have to wear a pad during her period, she had to wear Depends adult diapers as well. She had to know the location of the bathroom wherever she went. She could only shop in stores that had restrooms, which she would use when she got the store and then again before she left. She had to stop at gas stations all along her route whenever she traveled. Her lifestyle was upside down and she was always sad. She'd finally had it, she said, "I can't live like this anymore," and suggested the hysterectomy.

As I questioned Kimberly further, she told me that she had been on progesterone for five years. She started using it to prevent premature delivery (it stops uterine contractions) of her second child and had then continued using it for birth control. When I informed her that progesterone had been linked to depression, she was shocked and said, "I was never told that by any of my doctors." I always inform a patient when giving them progesterone for premenopause or menopause that it may make them sleepy. I ask them to let me know if they lose energy instead of boosting energy, and then we "tweak" the formula, dose, or time of day that it is taken. I gave Kimberly a 30-day salivary hormone test (see Chapter 9), which she took home and performed herself. It showed huge dips and plateaus in her cycle. I corrected it by prescribing varying doses of estrogen during the month (and small amounts of both progesterone and testosterone), along with a supplement designed to reduce excessive bleeding. Within one month she was no longer experiencing PMS, exhaustion (caused by the anemia she developed due to the huge blood loss), or depression. And, I am happy to report, she retained her uterus and ovaries.

In the same way that we as parents brace ourselves for our children going through their teenage years because of their hormones surging, we have to understand that perimenopause is the opposite of that. We're transitioning into a decline of our hormones. Fortunately, because of all the attention that's being given to hormone replacement and bioidenticals, this short period of our life is getting more attention, which is leading women to seek help before they reach menopause.

Perimenopause and the Fatigue Factor

When I talk about fatigue in relation to perimenopause, I'm talking about more than just being tired. I'm talking about a feeling of overwhelming, sustained exhaustion that decreases your capacity for both physical and mental functioning. It's a weariness that seems unrelated to the amount of sleep you get at night. It is a general lack of energy and motivation that is enough to interfere with your normal life.

Some of the usual manifestations of this kind of fatigue include:

❖ Always feeling run down and stressed

❖ Difficulty waking up in the morning

❖ Being dependent on coffee, tea, or high energy drinks for vitality

❖ Struggling to keep up with daily activities

❖ Not being able to bounce back from any illness or stress

❖ Lack of interest in sexual activities

❖ General feeling of weariness and discontent toward life

From Dr. Eva's Files

Jennifer is an attractive blonde, almost 44 years old. She has two children, one of whom is five years old, and another who is a year and a half. She came to me because she was experiencing several symptoms of perimenopause, which she described as "having horrible PMS all the time." Her periods, which were now coming every three weeks, were heavier than they used to be and very painful. She was experiencing wild mood swings, had gained weight, and was perpetually tired.

"My husband said, 'What is going on with you?' and I said it could be perimenopause. He said, 'How long is this going to last?' 'Could be five years,' I said. He sighed and said, 'Oh god. Five years . . .'

"Part of the problem is that I have two young kids, and I can't keep up with them. I'm okay in the morning, but by the middle of the day I feel like I can't function. I have to pick up my son from school at 2:00, and if I haven't had a nap, I can barely keep my eyes open. This happens every day. I go to bed at 8:30 at night, as soon as I put the kids to bed. I can't go out to dinner or anywhere else; I just don't have the energy. I've gained nine pounds in six months, even though my eating habits haven't changed.

"My poor husband feels incredibly neglected. I take care of the kids first. I try to take care of myself, which I'm clearly not doing a very good job of, and then whatever I have leftover is devoted to him. Which is virtually nothing. If I don't get some relief soon, my marriage might be over."

I checked out her hormone levels, and she was indeed in classic perimenopause with a low dip in progesterone. I cycled her with a topical progesterone starting on day 14 of her cycle up until day 28. She applied it twice a day. I also combined this with supplements including B vitamins, carnitine, EGCG, magnesium, and 5-HTP to help her get restful sleep. Within the first month she was back to her old self. She continued on that regimen until her transition into menopause.

When it comes to perimenopause, fatigue has its origins in hormonal imbalance, which can be due to poor nutritional choices, especially for women who follow low-fat, high-carbohydrate eating plans. These women often suffer from insulin resistance, which disrupts their bodies' glucose/energy metabolism. They get a burst of energy from eating refined, processed sugary treats, but quickly tire, and need to start the whole cycle again. Adrenal insufficiency due to stress, poor diet choices, or the effects of perimenopause on thyroid function can also lead directly to fatigue.

Hormone imbalances can also cause disrupted sleep, which often results in daytime fatigue. When you wake up in the middle of the night drenched in sweat, it's often difficult to get back to sleep. Erratic surges of estrogen can affect sleep cycles and make it impossible to get the deep sleep we all need to feel rested.

These estrogen highs and lows can also cause depression (a well-known source of fatigue). According to the ongoing observational Study of Women's Health Across the Nation (SWAN), in which 3,302 African American, Caucasian, Hispanic, Japanese, and Chinese women at seven U.S. sites have been evaluated annually since their enrollment during 1996–1997 at age 42 to 52, women with no history of depression are at sharply increased risk of first-ever, clinically significant depressive symptoms during perimenopause. This may be caused by low estrogen in the brain, which decreases neurochemicals such as serotonin, norepinephrine, and dopamine. For many women who go through this stage of depression, selective serotonin reuptake inhibitors (SSRIs)—antidepressant medications—can be very helpful because they increase the amount of serotonin available to the brain.

Is It Hot in Here?

You're sitting there watching TV or having a conversation with friends or maybe just looking out a window. Basically doing nothing, minding your own business. And suddenly it is unbearably hot in the room. You can feel your face and neck turning red. You begin to sweat. All you want to do is plop down into a chair with your face directly in front of a fan. Several minutes later, it's gone.

What was that? A hot flash. Although many women associate hot flashes with menopause, the truth is that they are one of the most common symptoms of perimenopause. For many women, the first symptom of perimenopause they experience is the hot flash, which is technically a vasomotor reflex (affecting the narrowing and widening of the blood vessels) that begins in the hypothalamus. In other words, the hypothalamus, which is sometimes referred to as the body's "thermostat," gets confused when estrogen drops. It makes the thermostat go way up into the red zone. The brain senses the temperature reading and immediately sets about trying to lower the heat. Your heart pumps faster, the blood vessels in your skin widen to circulate more blood to radiate off the heat, and you start to sweat to cool off even more—which can make you extremely uncomfortable, especially if all this is going on while you're out to dinner or in a business meeting. And then the heat, the flush, and the sweating are all compounded by embarrassment.

Some lucky women never have any hot flashes at all. Unfortunately, approximately 10 percent of women experience hot flashes for 10 years or more.

Another typical symptom of menopause is night sweats, which may be related to the fact that our bodies abide by a circadian rhythm. Over the course of a 24-hour day, certain hormones peak at certain times. Thyroid hormones and cortisol, for instance, tend to rise in the early morning. Night sweats are probably related to the normal changes in hormones that occur during sleep, predisposing or creating an environment where the hot flash can occur.

Treating Perimenopause with Hormones

Treating perimenopause with hormones is very similar to treating PMS with hormones. The first order of business is to have your hormones tested (see Chapter 9) to determine how much estrogen and progesterone you do or do not have. If your symptoms are severe and are interfering with your daily life, you may want to consider taking birth-control pills. These oral contraceptives can not only protect you against unwanted pregnancy, they can also relieve several symptoms of perimenopause, including PMS (which can sometimes get worse during perimenopause) and menstrual cycle irregularities. Birth-control pills can reduce or eliminate hot flashes and improve sleep problems and depression in most perimenopausal women; studies have shown that anywhere from 65 percent to 100 percent of women gain at least partial relief from hot flashes when using birth-control pills. It is not for everyone, however. Some women actually feel worse from taking the pill; they suffer from headaches or nausea, or it throws their hormones off in a wicked way. Also, there is a higher risk of side effects for women over 40 on birth-control pills, such as pulmonary embolism and deep vein thrombosis (especially if women are smokers).

Because of the sharp drop in progesterone, I usually advocate the use of topical progesterone during perimenopause. It's also the time I start adding testosterone because it increases energy and converts into estrogen. Some women need to take just progesterone or to cycle the estrogen with progesterone to keep the hormones higher while still allowing them to have their menstrual cycle.

THE THIRD PHASE: MENOPAUSE

- ❖ Are you experiencing hot flashes and/or night sweats?
- ❖ Do you experience short-term memory loss?
- ❖ Do you have difficulty concentrating?
- ❖ Are you experiencing vaginal dryness or pain during intercourse?
- ❖ Do you even care if you have intercourse?
- ❖ Do you suffer from insomnia?
- ❖ Have you noticed changes in the skin such as acne or facial hair?
- ❖ Are you losing your hair or is it thinning?

You know the drill. If you answered "yes" to two or more of these questions, you are probably experiencing the natural event known as menopause.

When all ovarian activity ceases, menstruation ends permanently. A woman has officially entered menopause when the menstrual cycle has not occurred for 12 consecutive months. Due to a decrease in hormone levels, namely estradiol, progesterone, and testosterone, the transition into menopause is often accompanied by an uncomfortable array of physical, mental, and emotional changes such as those mentioned above.

What is most important for women to remember is that hormone levels can be modified. You don't have to continue to suffer with PMS, perimenopause, or menopause just because they are natural occurrences. Our hormones change and are modified by our bodies literally from one day to the next. We now have many home tests available that allow us to measure hormone levels for an entire month to see where our deficiencies may be. What drives me crazy is when I hear women say, "My mother went through menopause, and she dealt with it so I guess I can deal with it, too. Eventually it will be over." Yes, it will. And so may your social life and your relationships with your children and your marriage, because you'll be a terror to be around. But you really don't have to live with it, deal with it, make the best of it, or anything else you may have heard about it. We are lucky that we live in an age when there are any number of solutions to the challenges brought about by moving into menopause.

This is a relatively new field in medicine. The main reason for this is that up until the early 20th century, women didn't often live beyond the age of 49. Therefore, menopause was quite a rare occurrence. Now, of course, women live 20, 30, or even 40 years after their last period. So women, along with their physicians, are still trying to figure out exactly what it takes to live out their later years with good health and great energy.

Menopause Around the World

In 2005, *The American Journal of Medicine* published an article called "A universal menopausal syndrome." The conclusion was that there was no such thing, as there were too many variables to take into account. That simply goes to prove once again that every woman's menopause is different.

Not only is menopause unique to every individual, it appears to have varying cultural connotations. Women in the West seem to have more menopausal symptoms than women in other parts of the world. In Japan, for instance, up until recently there was no phrase in their language for *hot flash*. Their word for menopause is *konenki*, which they define as lasting from their early 40s until their 60s. The end of their periods is just one aspect of these transitional years. There is no clear explanation as to why Japanese women report so few menopausal symptoms. Some researchers believe that their high intake of phytoestrogens (chemicals produced by plants that act like estrogens in animal cells) lessens hormonal imbalance, although no definitive answers have been found. Many cultures have an entirely different attitude toward menopause than we do. In both Chinese and ayurvedic medicine, the idea is not to treat a woman for menopausal symptoms; instead, it is to restore balance to the particular individual. Rather than being disturbed by the lack of libido caused by menopause, Bengali women think that sexual relations in older years is totally illogical. And many indigenous peoples, including rural Mayan communities in the Yucatán peninsula of Mexico, the Maori in New Zealand, and the Iroquois of North America, all believe that postmenopausal women are spiritual elders with considerable power and status.

Attitudes in many countries are changing, however, as what we know about menopause and how to treat it grows every year. We now know a lot more about how to deal with the changes in our bodies and any discomfort that comes along with getting older. That makes us different from generations of women who came before us, and gives us the opportunity to create new attitudes about our later years.

Symptoms of Menopause

Like PMS and perimenopause, the symptoms of menopause are highly personal. Every woman experiences this phase of her life in a unique way. Some women basically breeze through it. Most women experience hot flashes (approximately 80 percent of women in Western countries). Many women experience sleep disturbances. And a large number of postmenopausal women experience physical and mental exhaustion.

One thing we do know is that much of what happens during those postmenopausal years is due to the loss of estrogen (it doesn't completely disappear, but ovarian estrogen may decrease by up to 90 percent). Many aspects of our bodies rely on estrogen to keep them functioning properly, and that includes the mitochondria, those tiny energy centers of the cell. This appears to be especially true of the mitochondria in the blood vessels of the brain.

Many women complain that menopause has given them brain fog—they experience forgetfulness and a decline in verbal fluency (e.g., "I know I put that thing I bought yesterday in the, um, whatchamacallit, and now it's not there. And I can't find the um, um, thing that tells you how much it cost.") There is also a fair amount of data linking estrogen with a number of cognitive dysfunction and neurodegenerative diseases such as Alzheimer's and other forms of dementia. The brain is what we term sexually dimorphic, meaning that the brain develops one way under the influence of estrogen and another way if there is not as much estrogen present. If you look at some of the standardized testing of young children, girls and boys often test differently, which is thought to be due to the influence of sex steroids. Therefore, it is plausible that during menopause, when you have the withdrawal of estrogen, there may be neurological, psychiatric, and cognitive changes—which will show up more in some women than in others, due to genetic differences and sensitivities.

Menopause and the Fatigue Factor

In many instances, life does get harder as we get older. We have a lot to worry about—if our parents are still alive, we may be taking on more responsibility for their welfare. Now that women are having children later in life, many find themselves as part of the sandwich generation, having to care for both their parents and their kids. In a rocky economy, everyone experiences hard times. Add to that the fact that our bodies are having to work extra hard to try and adjust to all kinds of chemical changes, and it's easy to understand why women get so tired when menopause finally hits.

The biggest problem with fatigue is that it can prevent you from taking the necessary steps to fight fatigue! It's a catch 22. For instance, exercise is a particularly good tool to combat fatigue. But when you are so tired, exercise is the last thing on your mind.

Menopausal fatigue is different from drowsiness. With this kind of fatigue you don't necessarily want to take a nap—it's more that you don't want to do anything at all. It may be that you feel lethargic and lackluster all day, or it may come in intermittent spurts. And it affects both body and mind. You may often feel that you're just too tired to think clearly—or to think at all.

Once again, we can blame it all on changes in hormone levels. Hormones control energy at the cellular level, so when hormones decline dramatically (as they do in menopause), so does your energy. Of course, you have to add to this equation the fact that our REM sleep is often interrupted by hot flashes and night sweats during menopause, depriving us of a good night's sleep.

Treating Menopause with Hormones

I know that hot flashes and night sweats are uncomfortable. But I tell my patients to embrace them (that doesn't mean to keep suffering from them) as a sign of a new passage in their lives. These symptoms force us to look into our futures from a physical and an emotional point of view. It's a wake-up call. It means it's time to take time out of our day not only to think of ourselves as aging but

237

to do something about it in a thoughtful way. Otherwise, we may get arrested for ripping our shirts off in public before we sweat to death or get fired from our jobs for breaking into tears every half hour. I believe in hormone replacement when we need it. It not only relieves much of the discomfort that comes with menopause but also prevents us from aging faster than necessary.

Since we know that certain hormone production decreases when we hit menopause, we can easily conclude that this is a time when hormones are out of balance. That's why hormone-replacement therapy (HRT) came into practice. Then, in 2002, the Women's Health Initiative (WHI) report came out. It found that women taking HRT have a small increase in the risk of breast cancer, stroke, and dementia. This resulted in a huge backlash against HRT.

However, this study was conducted on women over the age of 64 who hadn't previously been taking hormones. This is not really a representative portion of women who need or choose to go on HRT. In addition, the women in the study were given Premarin with progestin, a harsh cocktail made from the urine of pregnant horses.

We have learned a lot since 2002. Now, women who choose hormone-replacement therapy are usually given a combination of estrogen and progesterone rather than progestin. This is because unopposed estrogen (estrogen without progesterone) can increase the risk of uterine cancer. In my practice, I never use progestin. I use progesterone either in a synthetic or a compounded bioidentical form. Long-term hormone therapy for the prevention of postmenopausal conditions is no longer routinely prescribed by many doctors. For some women, short-term HRT is exactly what they need to ease hot flashes, night sweats, and vaginal symptoms of menopause, such as dryness, itching, burning, and discomfort with intercourse. But what happens to you after you stop using those hormones? One thing is for certain: intercourse once again becomes painful, your skin turgor (elasticity) diminishes, and your brain doesn't work as efficiently, to name just some of the consequences of going without our natural-born hormones. Some doctors say that you should take the lowest effective dose for the shortest period of time. But I tell my patients to continue taking HRT for the rest of their lives. I really believe that hormone-replacement therapy is enormously beneficial for antiaging purposes and for general well-being. I put my patients on HRT indefinitely. It helps women both now and in the future.

The risk of developing cancer while on HRT is actually smaller than the risk of developing Alzheimer's or dementia by not being on hormones (a new study by Kaiser Permanente in 2010 showed women who start taking HRT in late life had a 48 percent chance of developing dementia, but women who started HRT in mid-life— around 48 years old—actually reduced their chances of dementia by 26 percent). And right now, while we do have a cure for many women with breast cancer, we do not have cures for Alzheimer's or dementia, so HRT may be the right way to go. When thinking about choosing synthetic HRT, factors to consider include your cancer history (women with a history of breast cancer should not take HRT), your age (younger than age 60 and within ten years of menopause is best), the intensity and frequency of your symptoms (20 hot flashes a day versus 2), and how much your symptoms interfere with your quality of life. We must approach whether to replace our hormones or not based on stratifying our risk factors for both taking and not taking (equally as dangerous for different reasons) our hormones. Nearly all women who have a mother with Alzheimer's and have done their homework insist on taking hormones for the rest of their lives.

Remember that estrogen also prevents osteoporosis, reduces cholesterol levels, increases the elasticity of the skin, helps prevent hair loss, helps prevent gingivitis and other dental diseases, helps protect against urinary tract infections and vaginitis, and helps us stay lubricated during intercourse (to mention just a few positive effects).

Another concern many women have about hormone-replacement therapy is weight gain. My patients are convinced that once they started HRT their weight increased. I try to educate my patients ahead of time while they are premenopausal to explain that the mere act of going into menopause will cause weight gain in and of itself. The degree of weight gain may escalate from the chemical estrogens and progesterones they are placed on, but it is rare for me to encounter a person on the appropriate HRT bioidentical whose weight has shifted upward. This is a complex subject matter, and unfortunately my editor has limited me to the pages already in this book.

Bioidentical Hormones

Just as every woman has a unique experience with PMS, perimenopause, and menopause, every woman also reacts differently to HRT. One of my patients came to me in an agitated state and said, "Doctor, you've got to help me. My internist recently started me on pharmaceutical HRT and ever since then, my appetite is out of control. I eat everything I see. If I see a woman across the street with a baby in a stroller, I literally want to run over there and eat that baby. Tell me, do I need to stop the hormone therapy?" I calmed her down and told her that no, she did not need to stop taking hormones. But I put her on bioidenticals instead of what she had been taking, and within days she was no longer agitated, she felt great—and her cravings were under control (no more cannibalism fantasies).

The good news is that there are now alternatives to synthetic HRT—they are called natural, or "bioidentical" hormones, meaning that they are biologically identical to human hormones. They are precise duplications of the estrogens and progesterone produced by the human female reproductive system. The molecular structure of these hormones—which are most often made from plants such as yams and certain nuts—is indistinguishable from that of natural hormones produced in the body. Because the body "sees" them as exactly like the hormones that are already there, they are less likely to cause adverse reactions.

Also unlike synthetic hormones, bioidentical hormones are tailored to your unique physiology and needs, and are prescribed for you by your doctor. When effects are known, the formulation can be fine-tuned or adjusted until you attain optimal relief. In my practice, I frequently recommend bioidenticals.

Bioidentical hormones come in various forms: creams, gels, patches, sublinguals (which are dissolved under the tongue), capsules, and vaginal applications. I particularly recommend the transdermal (cream) application, as the cream goes directly into the bloodstream and not through the liver, which can have potentially negative side effects.

Some women are mistrustful of bioidenticals because of the lack of long-term studies on their efficacy. Pharmaceutical companies are not interested in studying them because they cannot be patented. That means the big drug companies cannot make huge profits from them, which is why they have no interest in producing them, and in some cases are actively fighting against their having FDA approval. To me, the main concern is to be sure that the source from which they're obtained is maintaining quality control, which means more frequent testing so that the quality remains the same from batch to batch. Unfortunately, this may increase the price of the bioidentical, but it's worth it. After all, it is your body.

Remember also that pharmaceutical companies put a lot of additives into their products to extend their shelf lives. Many of these additives are heavy metals, which very possibly have long-term negative effects on the body. In contrast, bioidenticals have a shelf life of only a few months because they are natural and don't have additives and preservatives.

Bioidentical hormones are made at special pharmacies called compounding pharmacies. You should always get a recommendation for a compounding pharmacy from your doctor. To find a compounder who's accredited by the Pharmacy Compounding Accreditation Board, visit www.pcab.info.

From Dr. Eva's Files

Myra is a patient of mine who started having hot flashes when she was 53 years old.

"It wasn't just a hot flash," she said. "I felt as though my organs were burning inside. I felt that this must be doing permanent damage to my body. I also felt that with this type of internal combustion I should be burning thousands of calories and become very skinny. Well, neither the damage nor the weight loss occurred. I was up at least eight times a night and I was experiencing up to 30 severe, disturbing intense hot flashes. This was the norm, and it was very embarrassing in an extremely busy business world and social life. For two-and-a-half years I tried various methods and promises of relief. I came to you because of a recommendation from my daughter. You gave me a prescription for compounded hormones. You also gave me back my dignity and my peaceful sleep. It has been nearly two-and-a-half months, and I no longer have the horrible hot flashes I was experiencing. The special compounding of exactly what I needed did the trick. Manufactured meds just weren't performing."

THE PMS, PERIMENOPAUSE, AND MENOPAUSE
jump-start tips

Following are some natural treatments for PMS, perimenopause, and menopause. There will be some overlap as similar hormones are involved in each of these three stages, but my first choices for each stage are included here.

Natural Treatments for PMS

Several natural therapies are available for the relief of symptoms associated with PMS. Because every woman's PMS is different, some will work better than others. You may have to experiment with a variety of supplements until you find the one(s) that work best for you. These natural therapies are effective in most women because they address such factors as fluctuating serotonin levels, poor liver detoxification, cravings, and the synthesis of hormonelike substances called prostaglandins that cause inflammation. All of these factors influence the likelihood and duration of the symptoms of hormone imbalance. Suggested supplements include:

❖ **Krill oil:** Krill oil is a powerful source of omega-3 fatty acids. Studies have shown that after 45 days of taking krill oil, there was a statistically significant difference in both emotional and physical symptoms of PMS, including breast tenderness, joint pain, and dysmenorrhea (painful menstrual cramps). Krill are tiny crustaceans, known in Japan as the delicious delicacy *okiami.* Krill is also a traditional food of South Korea and Taiwan. Russia and Ukraine are also large markets for krill. Unlike fish oils, pure krill oil carries omega-3s in the form of phospholipids—liposomes or little packages that deliver the fatty acids directly to your body's cells.

❖ **Magnesium:** As discussed earlier, magnesium deficiencies can exacerbate several symptoms of PMS. Therefore, taking magnesium supplements can often improve these symptoms, which include mood changes, weight gain, swelling of the hands and feet, breast tenderness, bloating, and fatigue.

❖ **Chasteberry:** This herb, native to the Mediterranean, has been used for centuries in the management of gynecological complaints and is still popular for relief of PMS symptoms such as abdominal cramps, mood swings, depression, and fatigue.

❖ **5-HTP (5-Hydroxytryptophan):** The theory behind the use of this herb, derived from the seed of the African plant *Griffonia Simplicifolia,* is that it enhances levels of serotonin, which helps regulate depression, anxiety, and appetite.

❖ **Vitamin B$_6$:** A deficiency of this vitamin has been associated with decreased levels of neurotransmitters that control sadness and anxiety. Vitamin B$_6$ has been shown to relieve PMS symptoms such as depression, irritability, and fatigue.

❖ **Dong Quai:** This herb, also known as *Angelica sinensis,* is a plant that grows in Korea, China, and Japan and is traditionally used to relieve cramps and irregularity. Dong Quai is particularly useful in helping to end hot flashes and menstrual cramps. Note: dong quai contains coumarin derivatives, so anyone taking Coumadin, a prescription anticoagulant (blood thinner) that is also a coumarin derivative, should not take dong quai without the advice of a physician.

❖ **Evening primrose oil:** Evening primrose oil contains gamma-linolenic acid (GLA), an omega-6 essential fatty acid. Many PMS sufferers are found to have unusually low levels of GLA in their systems, which is why these supplements may help provide relief. By interfering with the production of inflammatory prostaglandins released during menstruation (prostaglandins are hormones that give us signals, such as pain and inflammation, that something is wrong), the GLA in evening primrose oil can help to lessen menstrual cramps.

❖ **Licorice (*Glycyrrhiza glabra*):** Licorice raises progesterone levels and has been known to ease certain symptoms of PMS, such as irritability, bloating, and breast tenderness.

❖ **Cramp bark (*Viburnum opulus*):** This herb relaxes muscle tension and spasms of the uterus, relieving menstrual cramps.

Natural Treatments for Perimenopause

Many of the same natural therapies that work for PMS will also work for perimenopause. In addition, you might try:

- ❖ **St. John's Wort:** This has been used as an herbal remedy and mood enhancer for hundreds of years. A little of this can even out your moods and help you feel normal once again.

- ❖ **Black cohosh:** This is an herb that can mimic what estrogen does in the body and reduce the incidence of night sweats and hot flashes, which can be particularly brutal.

- ❖ **Red clover:** This plant also helps with night sweats and hot flashes. To a lesser degree, tests are indicating that there may be improvements in bone health with this plant.

- ❖ **Evening primrose oil:** This particular supplement can be instrumental in reducing breast tenderness. Flaxseed and black currant oil are also in this category.

- ❖ **Valerian root:** This is an herb that has a sedating effect, and can be used by women who have sleep difficulties. Valerian helps elevate the amount of GABA in the brain, which calms the mind and body.

- ❖ **Ginseng:** This increases energy levels when suffering from fatigue. Many women report feeling revitalized while taking ginseng.

Natural Treatments for Menopause

Once again, many of the same natural therapies that work for PMS and perimenopause work for menopause as well. In addition, you might try:

❖ **Siberian rhubarb root:** Siberian rhubarb root has been recommended in Germany since 1993. It has been clinically shown to reduce menopausal hot flashes by 72 percent and significantly relieved other common symptoms including sleep disturbances, poor mood, and anxiety.

❖ **Vitamin E:** Some women experience a reduction in hot flashes when taking vitamin E. It is best to take three pills a day, one with each meal. Look for d-alpha tocopherol, which is natural vitamin E, and take no more than 200 IU at a time and never more than 800mg in a day.

❖ **Exercise:** I can't emphasize this enough: exercise is imperative as you get older, especially after menopause. Research shows that exercise alone can alleviate hot flashes. In one study, aerobic exercise reduced the severity of hot flashes in 55 percent of postmenopausal women. Regular weight-bearing exercise and strength training can help maintain strong bones, especially for women who choose not to take HRT.

❖ **Try acupuncture:** This ancient medicinal art can be useful for menopause as it works to release endorphins into the body which can help to improve the mood of menopausal women. It can also help to balance hormones and alleviate hot flashes.

❖ **Get a massage.** Massage is also useful as it helps to reduce the amount of stress that menopausal women suffer, and it helps to promote circulation. Better yet, get a dual massage with your husband or significant other for your sexual energy and to promote your health in every way.

Now that you've read through all but the last essential key to fighting fatigue and are following the Fatigue Solution program, you should be feeling reenergized and revitalized. If, for some reason you are not getting the results you want, turn to the next chapter and find out about some tests you can take to see if there are deeper problems you should explore further.

CHAPTER 9

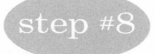

Have Yourself Tested

How can you know just what it is that is making you so tired? Especially if you've been to a health-care professional and they tell you everything's normal? The only way to know for sure is to go through a process of diagnostic testing.

These tests are usually done after you have already gone through several other channels. Most people first try to make lifestyle changes; they "clean up their act" by exercising more and/or eating a healthier diet. Not only do they find no relief, they usually fail at keeping up their good intentions. Then they visit one or more doctors, but get no answers that would explain their ongoing fatigue. That's when they are told that what they are experiencing is an inevitable part of aging and they should simply accept the way they feel as part of getting older.

The tests described in this chapter are for people who are not willing to listen to that advice. These are tests that you will not generally get from your general practitioner, but they are designed to uncover deficiencies in body chemistry that are preventing you from performing at optimal levels and from feeling your best every day.

You will probably have to ask your doctor about the specific test(s) you would like to have done. Don't be afraid to ask your doctor questions or suggest certain tests. When my patients do that, I always say, "Thanks for bringing that to my attention." I believe the more educated the patient is, the better the doctor can do her job.

These tests will help you help your doctor diagnose your problem and find the best treatment to get you back on track. Not every doctor is familiar with all the cutting-edge tests that are now available, and, unfortunately, HMO medicine doesn't allow for those doctors to freely order many of these tests. However, it is important that the doctor know about them so that he or she can order them if possible, or at least understand what they are so that you and your doctor can discuss the results if you get the test done elsewhere (some of these tests you can order yourself and do at home). The better the doctor is, the more open that doctor will be to your suggestions. Doctors are human beings; we can't know everything, but we can be open to learning.

Your doctor may be willing to order a particular test for you, or he may not think it's necessary. If you still want it done, another health-care professional may be able to get it for you. However, not many of these tests are covered by insurance, although some may be covered as out-of-network (services covered at a different rate) lab tests. You may have to pay for others out of your own pocket. This really depends on your insurance coverage, and you'll have to check with your company and your particular policy to be sure. You should always check with your health professional and your insurance company before you have these tests done so that you are not presented with an unexpected bill after the fact.

I've briefly listed eight of these tests here, as well as why you might want to have them done and what the results will tell you. If you think any of them might be helpful to you, you should discuss them with your doctor and/or your alternative health professionals.

There are a number of different laboratories my office uses for these various tests. For more information on these laboratories or for more guidance as to which labs would be right for you, check the Resource Guide in Appendix II or go to www.The FatigueSolution.com.

Food Allergies Profile Test

Why test: abnormal responses to food, including rashes, hives, asthma, eczema, itching, nausea, diarrhea, and fatigue

Food allergies can often result in decreased energy. It's important to rule out these allergies as the cause of fatigue and identify foods that may be causing health problems. Delayed food reactions can cause a multitude of seemingly unrelated health problems including IBS, fatigue, skin problems, joint pains, ADD/ADHD, and more. This test, called a RAST (radioallergosorbent test), measures the blood levels of Immunoglobulin G (IgG) antibodies in reaction to specific foods. Offending foods are typically milk, corn, and wheat and other gluten-containing foods. However, people are often surprised to find that it's not the milk they're allergic to, but something else they've been eating all their lives. People might find they are allergic to bananas or chicken or cinnamon or other very common foods.

Many people have skin tests done to measure food allergies. In this test, the surface of the skin is pricked or scratched, and a drop of the allergen in question is placed on the scratched skin. Skin testing to foods can give a sense, based on the size of the reaction, whether a person is truly allergic to the food, while a RAST actually measures the amount of allergic antibody to the food (or other substance, such as dog or cat hair or tree pollen). Skin testing doesn't always capture the allergies that a blood test can capture. Not to mention that a blood test can measure from 40 to 90 allergens at one time, which is not possible with skin tests (imagine having your back pricked 90 times in one sitting!). If a skin test and a RAST test agree, you can give the results even more weight.

Gastrointestinal Function Profile (Stool Test)

Why test: unexplained abdominal pain, diarrhea, constipation, or other gastrointestinal disorders and gas, bloating, or belching

As we know from Chapter 3, gut health is vitally important to our overall well-being. We need to be sure that we have the proper balance of bacteria in our gut so that we can easily digest our food, have efficient nutrient usage, and rid the body of waste and pathogens. Improper balance can lead to food allergies and sensitivities, as well as immune dysfunction, nutritional insufficiencies, mental and emotional disorders, and autoimmune diseases—all of which can in turn lead to energy loss and fatigue.

Every time we eat, we are exposed to a variety of organisms. Some of them are beneficial and some of them are harmful. Some are not harmful enough to cause major symptoms, yet they can still interfere with quality of life. The gastrointestinal function profile (GFP) can check for a wide variety of conditions and disorders, including inflammation, immune function, gluten sensitivities, yeast, pathogens, pancreatic function, and efficiency of digestion. It also tests for parasites and bacteria, as well as certain cancers. The test checks the PH balance of the gut to see whether you are effectively absorbing the nutrients your body needs. It checks for animal parasites or protozoa (one-celled organisms) growing in your gut (you can get protozoa from a dog or cat—they're not life threatening but they can cause discomfort and you do want to get rid of them). This is a much more varied and specific test than the standard type of stool test you would normally get from your gastroenterologist.

Adrenal Stress Index

Why test: excessive fatigue and exhaustion, waking up tired, inability to cope with stress, having low stamina, difficulty concentrating, poor digestion, or consistent low blood pressure

The adrenal stress index is a "spit test." Taken via saliva, it's the measure of an individual's response to stress. The test looks at DHEA-sulfate and cortisol. DHEA-sulfate is tested two times during the day and averaged. Cortisol is tested four times during the day and a rhythm is determined. We also look at the cortisol:DHEA-S ratio to help us determine your degree of adrenal stress. When cortisol levels are high, it usually means that there is chronic inflammation present in your body or that the mechanisms used by the body to lower cortisol are not functioning properly. When cortisol levels are very low, it is a sign of adrenal exhaustion or burnout.

There are stages of response to chronic stress and each stage impacts your health and hormones differently. The adrenal stress index allows you to identify your stage of adrenal fatigue or exhaustion so that you can optimally target nutrients and lifestyle recommendations to help you heal quickly and regain your energy. Once the tests have been interpreted (with the help of your health professional), you can actually change your response levels within several months and know exactly which supplements to take and when to take them, and which exercises and relaxation techniques you should perform.

HPA Profile

Why test: excessive fatigue and exhaustion, mood disorders, depression, anxiety, inability to concentrate, or insomnia

Deficiencies or imbalances in the main neurochemical pathways (the chemical processes of the nervous system) of the body can lead to a host of mood-related problems. If you are having problems with mood swings, energy levels, and cognitive functions, you don't have PMS and you're not perimenopausal, your thyroid is normal, but you can't get out of bed in the morning, you may be having problems involving the main neurotransmitters of the hypothalamic-pituitary-adrenal axis (HPA axis). In other words, your brain chemistry is not balanced. This simple urine and saliva neurotransmitter testing measures the ratios of serotonin, dopamine, GABA, and epinephrine (to name a few) and make it finally possible to treat mood imbalances (which greatly influence energy levels) through specifically targeted prescription medications or through nutraceuticals and supplements. In other words, this test can tell you (or your health professional) the exact pharmaceutical or nutraceutical you need to be on to get your neurotransmitters back into proper balance. This has the potential to dramatically change the way the medical profession diagnoses and treats mood disorders such as depression, anxiety, fatigue, irritability, and insomnia (to name a few) and a range of other neurotransmitter-related conditions.

Personalized FIT Genetics Profile

Why test: inability to lose weight

If you follow the Fatigue Solution philosophy and use the menu plan in Appendix I as a guide, you will lose weight. But if you have a target weight goal and you haven't quite gotten there yet, you might find yourself getting frustrated. That's when you might want to try the FIT genetics profile as a way to customize your diet and fitness program to your specific genotype (your genetic makeup). According to nutrition and fitness expert JJ Virgin, "Forty to seventy percent of weight gain is related to your genes and when you quit battling them and work with them, things get much easier." The FIT test (a simple spit test you can do at home) looks at 140 different genes to create your individualized weight-loss plan. According to Virgin, your genes play a role in your degree of appetite, how full you feel after eating, your need to seek out foods that you really want, your ability to not overeat in the face of stress or other triggers, your desire for sweets, and your need to snack. The FIT test suggests the type of diet and exercise on which you should focus to lose those last stubborn pounds.

Comprehensive Metabolic Testing

Why test: fatigue

There are several different versions of comprehensive metabolic testing, but they all basically measure levels of vitamin deficiencies, amino acids, oxidative stresses, and nutritional needs. This is the type of testing I used when I was working with a team from the Tour de France. I wanted to find the proteins each team member needed to maximize his energy and athletic capabilities. Before the testing, they were all using the same amino-acid powder to supplement their diets. With the help of the comprehensive metabolic panel (CMP), the team members were able to customize their diets to their indvidual needs, and went on to win the Tour.

This testing is important for all of us, because taking the wrong kind of amino acids can cause liver and/or kidney damage if used excessively. A CMP can be ordered through your doctor or through a nutritionist (and can also be ordered on my website, www.dreva.com).

30-Day Female Hormone Test

Why test: mood swings, lethargy, irritability, irregular periods, painful periods, uterine pain, craving sweet or salty foods, night sweats, hot flashes, or heart palpitations

If you are suffering from PMS or think you have a general imbalance of your female hormones, you might want to take the 30-day female hormone test. This is a home-based test you can order online. It is offered by several different companies. The test is designed to provide an evaluation of the sex hormones testosterone, progesterone, and estradiol. A kit is sent to your home, and you then collect between 11 and 13 saliva samples on particular days (the kit will tell you which days) in the privacy of your own home over a month-long period. This simple, noninvasive saliva test can determine levels and ratios of estradiol, progesterone, and testosterone. The reason the test is done over 30 days is that female hormones vary daily. In contrast, if you're testing for thyroid hormones, for example, there is not much variance from day to day or morning to night. If you're testing for cortisol levels, there is variation from morning to night, but not from day to day. There are, however, different amounts of estrogen and progesterone from one day to the next so the only way to know what is happening over a 30-day period is to test over 30 days. The test is useful for both premenopausal and perimenopausal women not currently supplementing with hormones. This test is especially useful in treatment of patients with chronic gynecologic disorders.

Intracellular Vitamin Analysis

Why test: overall feelings of fatigue or something being "not quite right"

In the beginning of this book, you read my story—how I was so run down and tired all the time and unable to find out what was wrong with me. Finally, I took a series of tests, including this one, that led me to the path of recovery. This is also the test that started me on my journey in integrative medicine. The intracellular vitamin analysis test by SpectraCell (www.spectracell.com) determines exactly which vitamins, minerals, amino acids, antioxidants, and metabolites an individual is lacking by analyzing his or her white cells through a sophisticated blood test (intracellular means inside the cell). The test also measures the cells' ability to withstand oxidative stress, which is responsible for chronic cell damage and disease.

By having a vitamin analysis done you will know your body's status with respect to many important vitamins and essential nutrients. You can be deficient in micronutrients and not even know it. Studies have shown that 50 percent of patients taking a multivitamin are functionally deficient in one or more essential nutrients that are vital to long-term health. Deficiencies suppress the function of the immune system and contribute to degenerative processes. So anyone who is interested in feeling his or her best can benefit from the test. Vitamin deficiencies aren't just a reflection of diet. Since we are all biochemically unique, nutrient deficiencies do not necessarily correlate directly with nutrient intake, even among those with similar health conditions. Many factors beyond diet determine whether nutrient function is adequate. These include biochemical individuality, genetic predisposition, absorption and metabolism, age, disease conditions, and medications.

The results of this analysis reveal your unique biochemical status as it relates to energy and endurance, cardiovascular function, antioxidant function, liver detoxification function, inflammatory problems including joints and skin, mental and emotional function, and digestive disorders. For example, this test might tell you that you are deficient in zinc (fatigue is one of the symptoms). In that case, nutritional supplements might be recommended, along with dietary sources rich in zinc, such as red meats, potatoes, wheat germ, nuts, and legumes. It is especially important that vegetarians get this kind of testing, as they are frequently deficient in amino acids.

Below is a sampling of the vitamins analyzed in this test, their functions, the symptoms of deficiency, and repletion information (sources for treating the deficiency):

Vitamin B$_1$ (Thiamin)

Function: B$_1$ is used by cells to make energy from the food we eat; it plays a crucial role in the metabolism of carbohydrates and proteins to produce energy for the body. Vitamin B$_1$ is also required for the metabolism of alcohol, so if you plan on drinking at all you'd better be sure your B$_1$ is in order. Because the heart, brain, and nervous system all require high levels of energy for proper functioning, vitamin B$_1$ is essential for the health of these body systems.

Symptoms: Thiamin deficiency can lead to loss of appetite, irritability, depression, mental confusion, fatigue, constipation, and nausea.

Repletion: Vitamin B_1 can be found in rice bran, wheat germ, pork, enriched grain and grain products (cereal), and legumes (beans, peas, soybeans, lentils). RDA is 1.0-1.5 mg per day for adults.

Vitamin B_2 (Riboflavin)

Function: B_2 is also helpful in metabolizing food into energy. One of its most important functions is that it helps the body effectively use all the other B vitamins. In addition, it works as an antioxidant fighting against free radicals (unstable oxygen molecules), is essential for red-blood-cell production, and, according to the U.S. National Library of Medicine (part of the National Institutes of Health), it is effective in reducing the number of migraine headache attacks in people who are prone to these kinds of headaches.

Symptoms: Riboflavin deficiency most often leads to depression and dizziness.

Repletion: Vitamin B_2 can be found in meats and dairy products, green leafy vegetables, and enriched grains and grain products. RDA is 1.2 to 1.8 mgs per day for adults.

Vitamin B_3 (Niacin)

Function: As well as helping metabolize food into energy, B_3 is effective in improving circulation and reducing cholesterol levels in the blood. B_3 is also important for adrenal health and is effective for people who are having sleep deprivation issues. There are two warnings I usually issue to my patients regarding niacin, however. One is that niacin can cause your capillaries to expand, resulting in a temporary reddening and itching of the skin. It only lasts a few minutes, but it can be annoying. The second warning is more serious. Niacin can raise blood-sugar levels, so if you have diabetes you should definitely consult your doctor before taking this vitamin (or any other vitamin for that matter).

Symptoms: Niacin deficiency most often leads to depression, muscular fatigue, indigestion, insomnia, and headaches.

Repletion: Vitamin B_3 can be found in meats, legumes (including peanuts), enriched cereals, and potatoes. RDA is 13 to 20 mg per day for adults.

Vitamin B_6 (Pyridoxine)

Function: B_6 is needed to metabolize proteins and is important for a healthy immune system, nerves, bones, and arteries. Additionally, it helps the nervous system send messages to and from the brain. As I also tell my patients who suffer from PMS, vitamin B_6 can help reduce bloating, breast tenderness, and premenstrual acne.

Symptoms: Vitamin B_6 deficiency most often leads to weakness, depression, irritability, insomnia, and anxiety.

Repletion: Vitamin B_6 can be found in meats, legumes, enriched cereals, potatoes, wheat germ, and bananas. RDA is 1.4 to2.0 mg per day for adults.

Vitamin B_{12} (Cobalamin)

Function: B_{12} is needed to form blood and immune cells, and support a healthy nervous system. B_{12} has many other benefits as well: it helps your body produce melatonin, the hormone that helps you get a good night's sleep; it can help diminish tinnitus (ringing in the ears); it helps produce serotonin, the neurotransmitter that keeps us feeling calm; and it is the major player in pernicious anemia, a deficiency in the production of red blood cells caused by a lack of vitamin B_{12}. Because B_{12} is found in animal-based foods, especially red meat, many of my patients who are vegetarians or vegans are deficient in this vitamin. They come to see me complaining that they are consistently exhausted even though they eat "clean and healthy." When I test them, I almost always find that they are lacking B_{12}.

Symptoms: Vitamin B_{12} deficiency most often leads to weight gain, fatigue, weakness, and irritability.

Repletion: Vitamin B_{12} can be found in animal foodstuffs. It is not found in plant foodstuffs. RDA is 2.0 mcg per day for adults.

Biotin

Function: Biotin is needed for proper metabolism of fats and carbohydrates. It also helps to strengthen skin, hair, and nails. I have had patients with persistent acne who come to my office because they've been to several different dermatologists, tried dozens of skin-care products, and have seen very little improvement. In fact, they are suffering from biotin deficiency. Once they start taking biotin supplements, they see a significant reduction in their acne problems.

Symptoms: Biotin deficiency most often leads to thinning hair, mild depression, fatigue, sleepiness, and muscle pains.

Repletion: Biotin can be found in egg yolks, liver, royal jelly, rice bran, legumes, whole grains, and fish. RDA is 30 to100 mcg per day for adults.

Vitamin C

Function: Vitamin C is required for several metabolic functions of the body. It is also necessary in the production of several stress-response hormones including adrenaline, noradrenaline, cortisol, and histamine. It is required in the synthesis of carnitine, an amino acid that facilitates the conversion of fatty acids into energy within the mitochondria. Vitamin C protects against heart disease in various ways; it enhances iron absorption, promotes excellent wound healing, and detoxifies the body by binding to certain heavy metals so that they can be eliminated from the body. One of its major roles is in the synthesis of collagen in elastin, the main structural protein of skin, cartilage, and blood vessels.

Symptoms: Deficiency symptoms include capillary fragility which often manifests clinically as bleeding gums, easy bruising, tender joints, muscle weakness, and poor wound healing. Subclinical deficiency (which means it may not be measurable) can also result in lowered immunity, anemia, and fatigue due to its role in carnitine and certain hormones.

Repletion: Vitamin C can be found in broccoli, Brussels sprouts, cantaloupe, cauliflower, citrus fruit, guava, kiwi, parsley, peas, potatoes, red and green peppers, rose hips, strawberries, and tomatoes. RDA is 75 mg per day for women, 85 mg per day for pregnant women, and 120 mg per day for lactating women.

Calcium

Function: The most abundant mineral in the body, calcium is needed as a component of hard tissue (bones and teeth) as a messenger that transmits hormonal information. It also aids in blood clotting, nerve impulse transmission, and muscular contractions. The most well-known reason for taking calcium is to help prevent osteoporosis. But I also recommend taking calcium for my patients who suffer from PMS, as it is very effective in relieving symptoms including depression, irritability, fatigue, abdominal cramping, breast tenderness, and headaches. In fact, a study published in 1998 in the *American Journal of Obstetrics & Gynecology* found that calcium supplementation produced a major reduction in overall symptoms associated with PMS.

Symptoms: Calcium deficiency most often leads to muscular and nervous irritability, muscle spasms, muscle cramps, and osteoporosis. Conditions known to decrease calcium uptake or distribution are decreased gastric acidity (meaning that when you take antacids, you are actually preventing calcium from being absorbed); vitamin D deficiencies; high-fat dietary intake; high oxalate intake (which you get from rhubarb, spinach, char, and beet greens); immobility; and psychological stress.

Repletion: Calcium can be found in milk, yogurt, cheese, bone meal, and canned salmon and sardines (with bones). RDA is 800 to 1,200 mg per day for adults. However, this dosage should be broken up so that you are taking the supplement twice a day because the body can't absorb more than about 600 mg of calcium at a time.

Chromium

Function: Chromium plays an important role in optimizing insulin function and in the regulation of blood-glucose levels. Chromium deficiency may be contributing to this country's obesity problem. Due to processing methods that remove most of the naturally occurring chromium from commonly consumed foods, dietary deficiency of chromium is believed to be widespread in the United States. Chromium deficiencies raise the likelihood of insulin resistance and lead to elevated levels of glucose, which can ultimately cause heart disease and/or diabetes.

Symptoms: Chromium deficiency can result in insulin resistance, high blood pressure, high triglycerides, high glucose levels, and high HDL cholesterol.

Repletion: Most foods provide only small amounts of chromium. Meat and whole-grain products, as well as some fruits, vegetables, and spices, are relatively good sources. No RDA has been established for chromium.

Coenzyme Q10

Function: CoQ10 is a powerful antioxidant, facilitating the removal of harmful free radicals from the mitochondria. It's an essential component in producing energy from oxygen. The heart especially depends on CoQ10 to maintain normal rhythm and to pump blood throughout the body. Many people who are on statin drugs (cholesterol-lowering medications) such as Lipitor, Mevacor, and Zocor have lower levels of CoQ10 because of the medication. Some doctors are now utilizing CoQ10 for treating congestive heart failure, morbid obesity, hypertension, and energy in general. Some studies have shown that CoQ10 may be useful in arresting Alzheimer's and in the treatment of Parkinson's disease. Many doctors are now utilizing it for treating congestive heart failure, morbid obesity, hypertension, and energy in general.

Symptoms: The most common deficiency symptoms are angina and fatigue, but may also include gingivitis (inflammation of the gums) and hypertension.

Repletion: The richest sources of CoQ10 are fish and red meat. The best sources of supplementation are soft gelatin capsules that contain CoQ10 in an oil base. Capsules range in dosages from 10 to 250 mg. Toxicity is not known, but doses greater than 250 mg can be associated with nausea and diarrhea.

Vitamin D

Function: Vitamin D is needed for healthy immune system development, and is essential for skeletal development and bone mineralization. Vitamin D deficiency can lead to osteoporosis. I advise any of my patients who are taking calcium supplements for bone strength that they need to take vitamin D as well, as it enhances the efficiency of calcium absorption.

Symptoms: Vitamin D deficiency most often leads to osteoporosis and decreased calcium absorption.

Repletion: There are only a few foods that are good sources of vitamin D, so vitamin D supplements are often recommended unless you are exposed to sunlight on your skin regularly. RDA is 200 IU per day for adults ages 19 to 50; 400 IU per day for adults ages 51 to 70; and 200 IU per day for adults older than 70.

Vitamin E

Function: Vitamin E is helpful for symptoms of menopause and is also needed for control of inflammation, red and white blood cell production, and connective tissue growth. It also works as an antioxidant against heart disease, cancer, and diabetes. Vitamin E is frequently added to lotions, creams, and other skin-care products because it has been shown to help the skin look younger by reducing the appearance of fine lines and wrinkles. Also, its antioxidant activity is quite valuable for aging skin, as it helps fight free-radical damage.

Symptoms: Vitamin E deficiency most often leads to muscle weakness and anemia.

Repletion: Numerous foods provide vitamin E. Nuts, seeds, and vegetable oils are among the best sources, and significant amounts are available in green leafy vegetables and fortified cereals. RDA is 15 mg per day for adults.

Folate (Folic Acid)

Function: Folic acid is needed to produce blood cells and other new tissue cells. It is essential for pregnant women, and women who are considering having children, to have enough folic acid. Taking folic acid supplementation before conception significantly reduces the incidence of birth defects known as neural tube defects (malformations of the spine and brain) such as spina bifida and anencephaly. Studies have also shown that women who consumed more folic acid had a significantly reduced risk of developing high blood pressure.

Symptoms: Besides being directly linked to birth defects, folic acid deficiency most often leads to fatigue, constipation, insomnia, headaches, memory impairment, and intestinal lesions.

Repletion: Folic acid can be found in legumes, enriched cereals, green leafy vegetables, wheat germ, seeds, nuts, and liver. RDA is 400 μg per day for adults.

Glutamine

Function: Glutamine is very important for energy, for the synthesis of protein, DNA, and RNA, and for removal of toxic substances. It is very useful in alcoholism and fatigue, because it helps remove toxins from the liver.

Symptoms: Glutamine deficiency most often leads to intestinal disorders and gastric ulcers. If you are fatigued, it may be helpful to take glutamine supplements.

Repletion: The best sources of glutamine are foods containing protein, such as milk and meats. No RDA has been established for glutamine.

Glutathione

Function: Glutathione is necessary for protection against harmful free radicals, for promoting the immune system, and as prevention for inflammation. It is produced by the body and found in every cell. It's often considered the preeminent antioxidant because it's found within the cell. It has potentially widespread health benefits because it is found in all types of cells, including the cells of the immune system, whose job it is to fight disease. It also helps remove toxins such as drugs and pollutants from the liver.

Symptoms: Some symptoms of glutathione deficiency are pain, muscle weakness, and fatigue.

Repletion: Glutathione is not well absorbed into the body when taken by mouth; therefore, it is better to take cysteine, which is a precursor to glutathione. Foods rich in cysteine are high-protein foods such as meat, yogurt, wheat germ, and eggs. Supplementation with up to 2000 mg per day of N-acetyl-L-cysteine is a safe way to take cysteine (which is not recommended as it usually poorly tolerated).

Inositol

Function: Inositol is needed for proper function of hormones. It also effectively promotes the body's production of lecithin, which helps move fats from the liver to the cells. This means inositol helps to prevent the accumulation of fats in the liver. It is sometimes used in the treatment of liver problems.

Symptoms: Inositol deficiency most often leads to eczema, hair loss, insomnia, and constipation.

Repletion: Inositol can be found in nuts, seeds, citrus fruit, cantaloupe, and organ meat. No RDA has been established for inositol.

L-Carnitine

Function: L-carnitine helps the body convert fatty acids into energy that is necessary for muscular and all other activities throughout the body. Because the main function of L-carnitine is to help the body burn fat into energy, L-carnitine supplements are commonly taken for energy boosts. For my patients who are trying to lose weight, I usually recommend they take L-carnitine with every meal and before they begin to exercise.

Symptoms: L-carnitine deficiency most often leads to fat deposits in the heart, which results in fatigue. Normal heart function depends on adequate supplies of L-carnitine. If the heart does not get enough oxygen, carnitine levels quickly decrease. The lack of oxygen leads to decreased energy production and increased risk for heart disease.

Repletion: L-carnitine can be found in red meat and dairy products; nuts and seeds; legumes; vegetables such as artichokes, asparagus, beet greens, broccoli, collard greens, mustard greens, and kale; apricots; bananas; whole wheat; wheat bran; bee pollen; and brewer's yeast. No RDA has been established for L-carnitine.

Magnesium

Function: Magnesium is vital for proper cell function, as well as for neuromuscular activity, energy metabolism, and membrane interactions. It is extremely important in the treatment of fatigue and is often associated with thyroid conditions. I recommend magnesium to my patients who suffer from migraines. I also suggest magnesium to help combat stress, improve adrenal function, and allow for muscle recovery.

Symptoms: Magnesium deficiency most often leads to fatigue, high blood pressure, vertigo, muscle spasms, poor wound healing, and bone loss.

Repletion: Magnesium can be found in nuts, whole grains, potatoes, legumes, and fresh vegetables. RDA is 280 to 400 mg per day for adults.

Selenium

Function: Selenium is needed for the activation of thyroid hormones. It is the messenger between the thyroid and the adrenal gland. Without selenium, you can have a thyroid that is functioning properly but still be exhausted because the thyroid and adrenal glands are not communicating with each other. Selenium is also essential for immune function and can help alleviate symptoms of heavy-metal toxicity.

Symptoms: Selenium deficiency is associated with a higher risk for inflammation and inflammatory diseases.

Repletion: Selenium can be found in wheat germ, bran, brazil nuts, red Swiss chard, whole-wheat bread, oats, brown rice, and turnips. RDA is 50 mcg per day for adults. However, in the presence of the iodine-deficiency goiter, selenium has been reported to exacerbate low thyroid function. In other words, if you give selenium to someone who is iodine deficient, it makes the hyperthyroidism worse.

Zinc

Function: Zinc is important in acid/base balance. It's a component of insulin, and it helps with energy metabolism and immune function. Zinc is also essential for combating hair loss, a complaint I get from many of my patients; it is estimated that female-pattern baldness strikes 10 percent of premenopausal women and 50 to 75 percent of women 65 years and older. This can be especially problematic for alcoholics (alcohol interferes with zinc absorption) and vegetarians, who don't get enough zinc in their diet.

Symptoms: Zinc deficiency most often leads to fatigue, dermatitis, acne, poor wound healing, decreased immunity, and hair loss.

Repletion: Zinc can be found in red meats, oysters, wheat germ, seeds, nuts, legumes, potatoes, and zinc-fortified cereal products. RDA is 12 to 14 mg per day for adults. Too much zinc can slow down hair growth, so do not take more than the recommended dosage.

Some of my patients who have taken the intracellular vitamin analysis test and then take the recommended supplements come back to me after several months and complain that they aren't feeling any better. Often, I discover that is because they are taking low-quality supplements. You can't just take any old vitamin and expect it to do a good job. Unfortunately, in this particular case, you get what you pay for. When a store advertises supplements on sale, it usually means that their expiration date is coming up quickly, and the store wants to get them off the shelf. The vitamins you buy from large chain stores often sit in your system for days, or come out in your stool as whole pills. Many of my patients say, "I take a multivitamin. Isn't that enough?" Usually, I have to say no, it is not enough. A multivitamin does not address specific problems they may have.

That's the reason I decided to create my own Abadi line of supplements (which you can find on my websites, www.dreva.com and www.TheFatigueSolution.com). I know that the ingredients in each product are of the highest quality. And if a particular product is not working for one of my patients, I know exactly what's in it and I can recommend something else that may work better for them, the same way your doctor might do if your medication isn't working as hoped. I am not saying that Abadi products are the only quality ones out there. But it's up to you to do your own research and be sure you are making the healthiest choices.

There are ways to determine which supplements are best. You can check the *NutriSearch Comparative Guide to Nutritional Supplements* (Professional Version) by Lyle MacWilliam, which was mentioned in Chapter 3. You can also follow these tips:

❖ **Check the expiration date.** Supplements lose potency over time. You don't want to buy the supplement that has the furthest expiration date, as that usually means it's been processed for a long shelf life.

❖ **Find out if your physician produces a line of supplements.** If a physician makes his or her own brand, it is usually as a result of many years of research. That is definitely true for my Abadi product line, which has been extensively researched and scientifically designed to deliver renewed energy.

❖ **Look for the USP (U.S. Pharmacopeia) Seal of Approval.** This is a reputable organization that tests vitamins and supplements to be sure that they contain what is on the label and that they don't contain any harmful contaminants.

❖ **Don't believe medical claims that are too good to be true.** The FDA doesn't allow manufacturers to claim that their supplement prevents or cures diseases. If a manufacturer claims that a supplement "cures cancer" or "prevents diabetes," for example, leave it on the store shelf.

There are several different reasons for testing. First, you can look at it from the perspective of antiaging. Overwhelming scientific evidence confirms that vitamin deficiencies are often associated with the overall condition of your health. Vitamin, mineral, and antioxidant deficiencies specifically have been shown to suppress immune function and contribute to arthritis, cancer, Alzheimer's, cardiovascular disease, and diabetes, not to mention fatigue. The testing I run gives me a past year's worth of nutritional evaluation on a cellular level, telling me what your body needs. If you're deficient in antioxidants, for instance, your cells are dying a slow death that is visible on your skin as accelerated aging. Even if you think you eat well, you may still be deficient. Micronutrient testing will help us determine exactly what you need.

When you've adjusted your lifestyle and balanced your hormones and given them a chance to recharge your body and you're still not feeling quite right, testing can tell you what modifications might still be needed. It can answer the question, "How can I maximize my body now so that I don't fall into a fatigue or disease state in the future?"

Testing can help you customize lifestyle changes to fit your particular needs. In a book like this, I can only make general recommendations that work for the majority of people. But I can't take your genetic, environmental, or behavioral history into account. That can be accomplished by taking one or more of the tests mentioned above.

Another reason for testing is that it gives a basis for comparison. For example, Helen, a 32-year-old single mother came to me to solve her fatigue issues. She claimed to be doing everything right—she exercised three to four times a week, she got a good night's sleep, she was enjoying a satisfying sex life, and she ate only in-season, locally grown vegetables and whole grains. I suggested she take the intracellular vitamin analysis test. As I suspected, the results showed she was deficient in several B vitamins. I recommended she take a B complex supplement. Six months later, she returned and was tested again. Not only did she state that her energy level was much improved, her test results showed that her deficiencies had been greatly reduced—which verified that we were on the right track for her recovery.

You know your body better than anyone else does. I hope that this book has helped you understand why you feel the way you do and what you can do to feel better. My goal is to help you generate physical as well as emotional strength by balancing hormones so that you can reclaim and restore your energy resources. I'm sure you are well on your way, and I wish you luck on your journey.

CHAPTER 10

Parting Thoughts: Getting Back to You

For me, reenergizing yourself is about optimizing the desire for life. It's about being able to do what needs to be done to take care of yourself and your loved ones. It's about taking pleasure in the small things as well as the large; it's being able to cope with the stresses of everyday life and being able to bounce back from the disappointments and failures that happen to everyone. It's enjoying today and looking forward to tomorrow.

Writing this book has been an incredible journey and an honor for me, and I hope reading it has been one for you, too. I hope that it has renewed your zest for life. I hope that it has enabled you to stand up for yourself and tell your health professionals that you will not accept anything less than their best efforts.

While you've come to the end of the book, you have not come to the end of your journey. This is just the beginning. Just keep going along the path you've started. If that old "F" word comes back knocking on your door, just shoo it away and keep following the Fatigue Solution program. Soon enough, your life will be back on track.

It's about being able to say, as many of my patients do, *"I got the old me back, and that's what I really wanted."*

I hope that this book has enabled you to do just that.

Don't forget to visit my websites (www.dreva.com and www .TheFatigueSolution.com) and the Resource Guide in Appendix II if you want to dig a bit deeper on some of the topics in this book. Also, please keep in touch and let me know how the Fatigue Solution program is working for you. I look forward to hearing from you.

Dr. Eva's Energy/ Fuel Matrix: Meal Plans and Recipes

designed by Samantha F. Grant, CN

Here's a myth buster for you: eating healthy foods does not equate to increased energy. For example, consider the following menu: breakfast—oatmeal; mid-morning snack—banana; lunch— tomato soup and two slices of whole-wheat bread; dinner—roasted vegetables and couscous. These are all healthy foods, but they do not produce the energy you need. In fact, eating those foods will initially increase your blood sugar, causing a surge of insulin. After the surge comes the familiar "crash" that happens when the insulin drops dramatically, causing hypoglycemia (meaning blood glucose, or sugar, drops below normal levels) which can trigger symptoms such as hunger, weakness, dizziness, shakiness, and sleepiness.

Unfortunately, when you are exhausted you often don't have the energy to make healthy choices. When I was going through my own bout with fatigue, I was eating all the time—and not eating well. I remember on one particular trip to Mexico with my husband, I could not stop eating. At one point, my husband said to me, in front of other people, "Would you please stop eating already?" which, needless to say, led to a huge argument that night. After blood analysis it was determined that the same deficiencies that were causing my sleep problems were also causing my sugar cravings. I began to change my eating habits little by little so that I was eating for energy.

Eating for energy is a protein-based food plan. All of the recipes (and snacks) included here were chosen for three reasons: they are protein-based, they are easy to cook, and they are low in calories. The sample recipes included here were contributed by nutritionist Samantha F. Grant, CN—as well as patients who are following the Fatigue Solution program (recipes denoted with an asterisk)—and were specifically designed with those criteria in mind.

What you will find in the pages that follow is a two-week eating-for-energy food plan. Each week is divided into three sections: suggested meals and snacks for seven days; a shopping list for the week; and recipes for each of the meals. The meals are not only healthy, they're delicious! You can follow the meal plans exactly as written, or you can mix and match. Most important, remember to have fun. Enjoy!

(*NOTE:* Unless otherwise noted, recipes make one serving. In the recipes that call for whey protein, I recommend my Abadi Beverly Hills Blend since I know the ratios and quality of the ingredients. Feel free to substitute any vanilla protein you prefer, but try to match the ratio of the ingredients for the best results.)

THE ENERGY/FUEL MATRIX DAILY FOOD PLAN

WEEK 1 MEAL PLANS

DAY 1

Breakfast: *Greco-Italian Scrambled Eggs*

Snack: 1 small apple with 2 teaspoons cashew or almond butter (all natural: no sugar or artificial sweeteners)

Lunch: *Shrimp Cobb Salad* with a slice of whole-grain, sugar-free bread

Snack: *Fruit Smoothie*

Dinner: *Veal Emince with Rice* and *Sautéed Spinach*

DAY 2

Breakfast: *Yummy Yogurt*

Snack: 12 almonds with 1 small peach or apple

Lunch: *Salmon Burger*

Snack: *Spiced-Up Toast*

Dinner: *Chicken Cacciatore over Polenta* with *Steamed Garlic Broccoli*

DAY 3

Breakfast: *Oats and Protein*

Snack: 1 tablespoon cream cheese with 3 celery stalks

Lunch: *Tuna Wrap*

Snack: 1 string cheese with ½ cup mixed berries

Dinner: *Halibut Tropicale* with *Asparagus Fries*

DAY 4

Breakfast: *Breakfast Parfait*

Snack: *3-Layer Dip* with 1 cup of veggies (bell peppers, radishes, sugar snap peas, jicama, cucumbers, or celery)

Lunch: *Chicken Waldorf Salad*

Snack: *Low-Carb Tortilla Wrap*

Dinner: *Broiled Filet Mignon* with *Roasted Veggies*

DAY 5

Breakfast: *Peach Pie Shake*

Snack: 1 cup of veggies (bell peppers, radishes, sugar snap peas, jicama, cucumbers, or celery) and 3 tablespoons hummus

Lunch: *Open-Faced Burger Melt* with raw veggie slices or small salad of mixed greens with a vinaigrette of 2 tablespoons balsamic vinegar, 1 tablespoon extra-virgin olive oil, and 1 clove chopped garlic

Snack: *Baked Apple with Yogurt Crunch*

Dinner: *Shrimp Sauté* with *Brussels Sprouts*

DAY 6

Breakfast: *Breakfast Sandwich*

Snack: 10 almonds, 1-ounce goat cheese, and 5 black olives

Lunch: *Kale Salad with Grilled Chicken*

Snack: 1 *Protein Popsicle*

Dinner: *Turkey Marinara "Pasta"*

DAY 7

Breakfast: *TBLAT*

Snack: *Spicy Deviled Eggs*

Lunch: *Chicken Caesar*

Snack: 1 small apple with 2 teaspoons cashew or almond butter (all natural: no sugar or artificial sweeteners)

Dinner: *Meatloaf* and *Faux Tatoes*

WEEK 1 SHOPPING LISTS

Proteins:

Alaskan salmon (canned)

Almonds

Black beans (organic canned)

Chicken breasts (boneless and skinless)

Chunk light tuna (canned in water)

Eggs

Filet mignon

Ground beef (97% lean, organic, grass fed if possible)

Ground turkey (white meat)

Halibut fillets

Hummus

Pine nuts

Shrimp

Turkey bacon

Turkey sausage patties

Veal

Walnuts

Whey protein powder (vanilla and chocolate)

Cheese and Milk:

Almond butter (all natural)

Almond milk

Blue cheese

Brie cheese

Butter

Coconut milk (organic, light)

Cream

Cream cheese

Feta cheese

Goat cheese

Milk (whole, organic)

Parmesan cheese (grated)

Swiss cheese

Yogurt (whole plain and 2% Greek)

Fruits and Vegetables:

Apples (Granny Smith plus a variety of small apples)

Asparagus

Avocado

Baby spinach

Banana

Berries (mixed, fresh, or frozen)

Broccoli florets

Brussels sprouts

Cauliflower

Celery

Cherries (dried)

Cucumber

Cranberries (dried)

Garlic

Grapes (red)

Jicama

Kale (dinosaur or black)

Lemon

Mango

Mixed greens

Olives (black)

Onions (red, white, and green)

Peaches (fresh and frozen)

Pepper (red and green)

Radishes

Romaine lettuce

Sugar snap peas

Sweet potato

Tomato (plum and Roma)

Zucchini

Breads and Grains:

Bread (sliced, whole-grain, sugar-free)

Breadcrumbs (whole-grain)

Cereal (whole-grain)

Croutons (whole-grain)

English muffins (Ezekiel or whole-grain)

Flour (almond flour preferred)

Hamburger buns (Ezekiel or whole-grain)

Pasta (brown-rice or whole-grain)

Polenta (premade)

Rice (brown)

Steel cut oats

Tortillas (low-carb, whole-grain, spelt, or Ezekiel)

Condiments and Spices:

Agave nectar

Balsamic vinegar

Basil (fresh and dried)

Black pepper

Caesar salad dressing (low-fat)

Chili powder

Cinnamon

Dijon mustard

Dry white vermouth

Flaxseed (ground)

Fruit spreads (all natural)

Garlic powder

Garlic salt

Ginger (ground)

Grapeseed oil

Honey mustard salad dressing (low-fat)

Ketchup

Lecithin

Lemon pepper

Mayonnaise (low-fat, canola)

Olive oil

Oregano (dried)

Pasta sauce (organic)

Pumpkin-pie spice

Salsa

Salt

Sea salt

Stevia

Thyme

Tomato paste

Vanilla extract

Vermouth

White cooking wine

Xylitol

WEEK 1 RECIPES

<u>DAY 1</u>

GRECO-ITALIAN SCRAMBLED EGGS*

3 eggs (2 egg whites and 1 whole egg or 4 egg whites)
1 tablespoon organic whole milk
⅛ teaspoon salt
½ small Roma tomato, chopped
1 teaspoon olive oil
2 teaspoons crumbled feta cheese
2–3 large basil leaves, snipped
Salt and pepper, to taste

In a bowl, beat eggs, milk, and salt until frothy. In a small frying pan, heat olive oil on medium to medium-high heat until pan is hot, then pour in the egg mixture. Cook eggs, stirring occasionally until halfway cooked, then add chopped tomatoes. Cook all the way through and then stir in feta and basil. Makes 2 servings.

SHRIMP COBB SALAD*

2 cups romaine lettuce, cut into bite-size pieces
1 tablespoon low-fat honey mustard dressing
1 hard-boiled egg, cubed
½ avocado, cut into small chunks
6–8 steamed shrimp, peeled and cut into bite-size pieces
1 tablespoon crumbled blue cheese

In a large bowl, mix lettuce with dressing. Place egg, avocado, shrimp, and blue cheese on top. Toss together. Makes 2 servings.

FRUIT SMOOTHIE*

½ cup organic whole milk

½ teaspoon vanilla extract

½ cup frozen fruit or fresh fruit (strawberries, blueberries, etc.) or ½ banana

4–5 ice cubes

2 scoops whey protein powder (1 serving according to your protein powder mix)

2 teaspoons lecithin

1–2 teaspoons xylitol or stevia (optional)

Pour milk, vanilla, frozen or fresh fruit, ice cubes, protein powder, and lecithin in blender. Pulse twice for 5 seconds each time then puree until smooth. Sweeten with xylitol or stevia if desired. Makes 2 servings.

VEAL EMINCE WITH RICE*

1 cup brown rice

8 ounces veal

1 clove of garlic, finely chopped

½ yellow onion, coarsely chopped

2 teaspoons olive oil

¼ cup flour (almond flour preferred)

½ cup white cooking wine (sauvignon blanc or chablis)

1 tablespoon of cream (optional)

Salt and pepper to taste

Cook rice according to directions on package.

While rice is cooking, slice veal into ¼-inch thick strips. In a small sauté pan, sauté onion and garlic with olive oil until soft. Toss veal in flour. Add floured veal to sauté mixture and cook combination on medium-high heat until veal is lightly golden. Add wine to pan and bring to boil. Cook for about 3–5 minutes at boil then lower heat to simmer, add cream and mix thoroughly. Cook uncovered until veal is cooked through medium rare to well done, according to your preference. Stir frequently while cooking. Serve over rice. Makes 2 servings.

SAUTÉED SPINACH

1 teaspoon olive oil
1 clove garlic, chopped
2 cups washed baby spinach
Pinch of salt

In skillet, heat olive oil and garlic on medium heat until garlic is golden (do not overcook garlic or it will be bitter). Add spinach and 1 teaspoon of water. Stir. Cook spinach until wilted. Makes 2 servings.

DAY 2

YUMMY YOGURT

1 cup whole plain yogurt
2 teaspoons xylitol
1 teaspoon vanilla extract
½ cup sliced or cubed fruit of your choice

Mix all ingredients together and eat.

SALMON BURGERS*

One 10-ounce can Alaskan salmon
2 tablespoons lemon juice
1½ teaspoons Dijon mustard
¾ cup dry whole-grain breadcrumbs
½ cup sliced green onions
3 egg whites
4 Ezekiel or whole-grain hamburger buns
4 leaves of romaine lettuce
4 tomato slices

Drain salmon, combine lemon juice and mustard. Blend salmon with breadcrumbs, green onions, and lemon juice mixture. Mix in egg whites. Form mixture into 4 patties and grill or broil until golden brown and heated through. Serve each burger on a bun with lettuce, tomato slices, and condiments as desired. Makes 4 servings.

SPICED-UP TOAST

Three 1-ounce slices of Brie cheese
2 slices whole-grain, sugar-free bread, toasted
2 teaspoons of all-natural fruit spread (fig, raspberry, strawberry, etc.) or fresh fruit if you prefer

Place 1½ slices of Brie on each slice of toast and top with fruit spread. Makes 2 servings.

CHICKEN CACCIATORE OVER POLENTA

Two 2-inch-thick slices of polenta
1 teaspoon olive oil
½ clove of garlic, chopped
¼ yellow onion, chopped
1 boneless skinless chicken breast cut in half lengthwise
1 tablespoon of flour (almond flour preferred)
1 plum tomato cubed
¼ cup of white cooking wine
1 teaspoon of dry white vermouth
Salt to taste
Pinch of oregano

Prepare polenta according to directions on package.

In small frying pan, heat oil, garlic, and onions over medium heat until soft. Place chicken breast in flour, lightly flouring on both sides. Place floured chicken in frying pan and lightly brown with the onion mixture. Once chicken is browned, add tomato and cook for 10–15 minutes, then add wine, vermouth, salt, and oregano. Bring to a boil, then lower heat to low. Cook until chicken is fully cooked, approximately 15 minutes. Place chicken mixture over polenta.

STEAMED GARLIC BROCCOLI

1 cup broccoli florets
Garlic salt, to taste
1 teaspoon olive oil
¼ lemon

Steam broccoli to your liking. Once cooked, remove and place in bowl. Sprinkle with garlic salt, drizzle olive oil, and squeeze lemon over the top. Toss until mixed.

<u>DAY 3</u>

OATS AND PROTEIN

½ cup steel-cut oats
2 tablespoons vanilla whey protein powder
1 teaspoon ground flaxseed
¼ teaspoon cinnamon
½ teaspoon xylitol
¼ cup organic whole milk

Cook the oats as instructed on the package. Once cooked, mix in the remaining ingredients.

TUNA WRAP

1 can chunk light tuna in water, drained
1 teaspoon canola mayo
1 teaspoon dried cranberries
1 teaspoon diced red onion
Lemon pepper
1 tortilla (whole Spelt, Ezekiel, or whole-grain)
1 cup mixed greens
¼ cup chopped Roma tomatoes

Mix tuna, mayo, cranberries, onion, and lemon pepper together. Spread mixture on tortilla and top with greens and tomatoes. Wrap and serve.

HALIBUT TROPICALE

1 teaspoon grapeseed oil
Two 5-ounce halibut fillets
½ teaspoon sea salt
½ teaspoon lemon pepper
1 teaspoon agave nectar
2 tablespoons chunky salsa
2 teaspoons chopped mango

Preheat oven to 350 degrees. Line small baking dish with 1 teaspoon grapeseed oil. Place fish in dish skin side down. Season with salt and lemon pepper, drizzle with agave. Cover and place in oven. Cook for 15 minutes and top with salsa and mango. Makes 2 servings.

ASPARAGUS FRIES

1 pound fresh asparagus, trimmed
1 tablespoon grapeseed or olive oil
½ teaspoon garlic salt
1 teaspoon grated Parmesan cheese

Preheat the oven to 350 degrees. Toss asparagus in oil and garlic salt. Spread evenly on baking sheet and cook for 10 minutes at 350 degrees. Toss with Parmesan cheese and serve. Makes 2 servings.

DAY 4

BREAKFAST PARFAIT

1 cup 2% Greek yogurt
1 cup mixed berries, fresh or frozen
3 tablespoons whole-grain cereal

In a tall glass, make a layer with half of the yogurt, then create a layer with half of the fruit, then make a layer with half of the cereal. Repeat with remaining ingredients.

3-LAYER DIP

½ cup pureed organic canned black beans
½ avocado, smashed
½ cup salsa

Spread beans on a plate and top with avocado and salsa.

CHICKEN WALDORF SALAD

1 stalk celery, chopped
1 tablespoon low-fat canola mayo or 2% Greek yogurt
¼ teaspoon thyme
¼ teaspoon oregano
½ lemon, squeezed
4 ounces grilled chicken, chopped
1 tablespoon chopped walnuts
6 red grapes
2 tablespoons chopped green apple
2 cups mixed greens

Mix celery, mayo, thyme, oregano, and lemon juice in a small bowl. Add chicken. Mix well and add a little water if too dry. Top mixed greens with mayo-chicken mix and garnish with apple, walnuts, and grapes. Add more lemon, if desired.

LOW-CARB TORTILLA WRAP

2 teaspoons all-natural almond butter
1 tortilla (whole-grain or Ezekiel)
1–2 tablespoons of chopped green apple

Spread almond butter on tortilla and fill with chopped apples. Wrap and serve.

BROILED FILET MIGNON

One 4-ounce filet, 1- to 2-inches thick
1/8 teaspoon salt
1/8 teaspoon black pepper, coarsely ground
1 teaspoon butter

Preheat oven to broil. Sprinkle filet with salt and black pepper and place on broiler rack. Spread ½ teaspoon butter on filet and broil for about 8 minutes. Use remainder of butter on filet when you turn it. Broil to preferred doneness and serve.

ROASTED VEGGIES

1 cup asparagus, trimmed
1 cup Brussels sprouts, trimmed and cut in half
1 small sweet potato (skin on)
2 teaspoons grapeseed oil
¼ teaspoon sea salt
¼ teaspoon black pepper

Preheat oven to 450 degrees. Place all vegetables in a bowl and add grapeseed oil, salt, and pepper. Spread potatoes and Brussels sprouts evenly on baking sheet and roast for 15 minutes. Add asparagus and roast an additional 15 minutes, turning vegetables as needed.

DAY 5

PEACH PIE SHAKE

4 ounces light coconut milk
4 ounces water
1 scoop vanilla whey protein powder
½ cup frozen peaches
¼ teaspoon cinnamon
¼ teaspoon ground ginger
½ teaspoon xylitol

Blend all ingredients until smooth.

OPEN-FACED BURGER MELT

4 ounces lean ground beef (97%) organic, grass-fed if possible
1 slice Swiss cheese
½ hamburger bun (Ezekiel or whole-grain)
1 romaine lettuce leaf
1 slice tomato
1 slice onion

Form beef into a patty, and cook until desired doneness. Add cheese immediately after cooking. Place on half bun. Top with lettuce, tomato, and onion.

BAKED APPLE WITH YOGURT CRUNCH

1 Granny Smith apple
½ teaspoon pumpkin pie spice
1 teaspoon xylitol
1 tablespoon Greek yogurt
1 tablespoon ground flaxseed

Preheat oven to 350 degrees. Peel and chop apple. Combine with pumpkin pie spice and xylitol. Bake for 20 minutes. Top with Greek yogurt and flaxseed.

SHRIMP SAUTÉ

10 medium shrimp
1 tablespoon butter
1 clove garlic
¼ teaspoon lemon pepper

Peel and devein shrimp. Heat butter over medium-high heat, adding garlic and lemon pepper. Add shrimp and sauté for 6 minutes or until shrimp are a deep pink color.

BRUSSELS SPROUTS

2 cups Brussels sprouts
2 teaspoons grapeseed oil
2 tablespoons chopped red onion
¼ teaspoon salt
¼ teaspoon lemon pepper
⅓ cup water

Peel off outside leaves of Brussels sprouts. Cut off stalk and cut in half. Heat oil in skillet over medium-high heat. Sauté onion for 2 minutes, or until softened. Add Brussels sprouts, salt, and lemon pepper. Sauté at high heat for 1 minute, tossing mixture constantly. Add water and reduce heat to low. Cover and simmer until Brussels sprouts are al dente, approximately 15 minutes, checking to make sure water does not cook off. Serves 2.

DAY 6

BREAKFAST SANDWICH

1 turkey sausage patty
1 egg
1 slice Swiss cheese
1 slice tomato
½ Ezekiel or whole-grain English muffin

Cook sausage patty as directed on package. Beat and scramble egg. Assemble all ingredients on English muffin and serve.

KALE SALAD WITH GRILLED CHICKEN

1 head of dinosaur or black kale
1 tablespoon olive oil
1 lemon, juiced
2 tablespoons warm water

Dash of stevia or xylitol powder
1 tablespoon pine nuts
1 tablespoon dried cherries
Sea salt, to taste
1 teaspoon goat cheese
4 ounces grilled chicken strips

Take kale off stalk and place in large bowl. Set aside. In small bowl, combine oil, lemon juice, water, and stevia or xylitol powder. Pour liquid mixture over kale and add pine nuts, cherries, and salt. Mix well. Allow to marinate in fridge for 30 minutes. Add goat cheese and toss before serving. Top with chicken. Without the chicken strips, this salad can be served alongside any protein as a complete meal.

PROTEIN POPSICLE

1½ cups unsweetened coconut or unsweetened almond milk
1 cup frozen berries
1 scoop vanilla whey protein powder
1 teaspoon xylitol

Place all ingredients in blender and pulse until mixed, then pour into popsicle molds and freeze.

TURKEY MARINARA "PASTA"

8 ounces ground white turkey meat
1 teaspoon grapeseed oil
¼ teaspoon chili powder
2 tablespoons chopped red onion
2 tablespoons chopped red pepper
¼ teaspoon dried basil
¼ teaspoon dried oregano
¼ teaspoon garlic powder
One 22-ounce jar organic pasta sauce

2 cups steamed broccoli
2 cups steamed zucchini or other mixed green veggies
½ cup brown rice pasta, cooked
2 teaspoons goat cheese

Brown turkey in skillet with grapeseed oil and chili powder, onion, pepper, basil, oregano, and garlic powder. Mix in pasta sauce. Cover and allow to simmer for 30–40 minutes. Meanwhile, steam veggies and cook pasta according to package. Drain pasta and top with veggies, turkey marinara sauce, and goat cheese. Makes 2 servings.

<u>DAY 7</u>

TBLAT

3 slices turkey bacon
⅓ avocado
1 slice whole-grain, sugar-free toast
1 small tomato, sliced
2 romaine lettuce leaves

Cook turkey bacon. Smash avocado and spread onto toast. Top with tomatoes and lettuce.

SPICY DEVILED EGGS

2 eggs
1 teaspoon canola mayo
1 teaspoon Dijon mustard
⅓ teaspoon sea salt

Hard-boil eggs. When done, cut in half lengthwise, gently removing the yolks. Smash yolks and combine them with mayo, mustard, and salt. Spoon mixture into whites.

CHICKEN CAESAR

5 ounces grilled chicken breast
2 cups romaine lettuce
5 whole-grain croutons
2 teaspoons grated Parmesan cheese
2 teaspoons bottled low-fat Caesar dressing

Combine all ingredients and toss until well mixed.

MEATLOAF

1 pound lean ground beef (97%) organic, grass fed if possible
1 small yellow onion, chopped
½ teaspoon chili powder
½ teaspoon dried basil
½ teaspoon dried oregano
½ teaspoon garlic powder
One 6-ounce can tomato paste
½ cup of fresh whole-grain breadcrumbs
1 egg
⅓ cup ketchup
⅓ cup balsamic vinegar
1 teaspoon xylitol

Preheat the oven to 350 degrees. Brown ground beef with onion and spices in nonstick skillet. When done, add tomato paste and transfer to bowl. Mix in breadcrumbs and egg. Put all ingredients a loaf pan and cook for 35 minutes. Combine ketchup, balsamic vinegar, and xylitol in small bowl. Spread over meatloaf and cook an additional 10 minutes. Makes 3–4 servings.

FAUX TATOES

1 large head of cauliflower, trimmed
½ teaspoon sea salt

1 teaspoon butter

Steam cauliflower until soft. Place in large bowl, add sea salt and butter. Puree mixture with a hand held blender until smooth. Makes 3–4 servings.

WEEK 2 MEAL PLANS

DAY 8

Breakfast: *Chocolate Strawberry Shake*

Snack: 4 whole-grain crackers with 1 tablespoon all-natural almond butter

Lunch: *Salmon Nicoise Salad*

Snack: 1 small apple with 2 ounces goat cheese

Dinner: *Broiled Top Sirloin* with *Roasted Butternut Squash* and 1 cup steamed broccoli with 1 teaspoon olive oil

DAY 9

Breakfast: *Protein Pancakes*

Snack: *Chocolate Pudding*

Lunch: *Mediterranean Chicken Burger,* 1 cup carrots and/or jicama with 1 tablespoon hummus

Snack: 1 tablespoon of cream cheese split between 2 celery sticks, top each with 6 dried cranberries

Dinner: *Italian Turkey Sausage Stir Fry*

DAY 10

Breakfast: *Veggie Omelet*

Snack: 1 ounce goat cheese with ½ cup fresh berries

Lunch: *Oriental Chicken Wrap*

Snack: 12 almonds and 1 small apple

Dinner: *Turkey Black Bean Chili* with small salad of mixed greens with a vinaigrette of 2 tablespoons balsamic vinegar, 1 tablespoon extra-virgin olive oil, and 1 clove chopped garlic

DAY 11

Breakfast: 2 turkey sausage links, 1 slice whole-grain, sugar-free toast with 1 teaspoon goat cheese and 1 teaspoon sugar-free fresh fruit preserves

Snack: Abadi Beverly Hills Bar or another protein bar that contains no soy, sugar, or artificial sweeteners and has fewer than 200 calories

Lunch: leftover *Turkey Black Bean Chili* with small salad of mixed greens with a vinaigrette of 2 tablespoons balsamic vinegar, 1 tablespoon extra-virgin olive oil, and 1 clove chopped garlic

Dinner: premade roasted chicken, *Butternut Squash Soup,* small salad of mixed greens with a vinaigrette of 2 tablespoons balsamic vinegar, 1 tablespoon extra-virgin olive oil, and 1 clove chopped garlic

DAY 12

Breakfast: 2 *Chocolate Protein Muffins* with 2 teaspoons all-natural almond butter

Snack: *Pumpkin Yogurt*

Lunch: *Turkey Roll-Ups* with *Lentil Soup*

Snack: *Vanilla Strawberry Shake*

Dinner: *Broiled Filet Mignon, Sautéed Spinach,* and *Roasted Rosemary Potatoes*

DAY 13

Breakfast: *South-of-the-Border Scramble*

Snack: 12 almonds, 1 organic pear

Lunch: *Mini Pizzas* with small salad of mixed greens with a vinaigrette of 2 tablespoons balsamic vinegar, 1 tablespoon extra-virgin olive oil, and 1 clove chopped garlic

Snack: ½ cup 2% cottage cheese and ½ cup blueberries

Dinner: *Tuna Pasta*

DAY 14

Breakfast: *Sweet Potato Pie Protein Shake*

Snack: 3 tablespoons *White Bean Dip,* 10 raw baby carrot sticks

Lunch: *Curried Tuna Salad*

Snack: *Almond Butter Delight*

Dinner: *Super Supper Scramble*

WEEK 2 SHOPPING LISTS

(NOTE: Items from Week 1 that will probably be left over have not been repeated, especially where condiments and spices are concerned.)

Proteins:

Abadi Beverly Hills Fiber Blend (or ground chia or ground flax)

Black beans (organic canned)

Chicken (premade, roasted)

Chicken breasts (bonelesss and skinless)

Chunk light tuna (canned in water)

Deli turkey (low-sodium)

Eggs

Filet Mignon

Ground chicken (white meat)

Ground turkey (white meat)

Hummus

Lentils (canned or dry)

Pinto beans (organic canned)

Salmon filets (preferably wild)

Turkey sausage links

Whey powder (vanilla and chocolate)

White beans (canned or dry)

Cheese and Milk:

Almond milk (unsweetened vanilla and chocolate)

Coconut milk (organic, light)

Cotija cheese (white cheese)

Cottage cheese (2%)

Cream cheese

Feta cheese

Goat cheese

Mozzarella cheese (part-skim)

Ricotta cheese

Fruits and Vegetables:

Apples

Asparagus

Avocado

Berries (mixed, fresh)

Blueberries (fresh)

Broccoli

Butternut squash

Carrots (baby and regular)

Caulifower

Celery

Cranberries (dried)

Green beans (fresh)

Jalapeños

Jicama

Lemon

Mandarin oranges

Mango

Mixed greens

Onions (red and white)

Peppers (red and yellow)

Potatoes (large white and small red)

Pumpkin puree

Raisins

Spinach (fresh)

Strawberries (frozen)

Sundried tomatoes

Sweet potato

Tomatoes (canned, chopped and fresh)

Zucchini

Breads and Grains:

Bread (sliced, whole-grain, sugar-free)

Flaxseed meal

Pancake mix (gluten-free)

Hamburger buns (Ezekiel or whole-grain)

Pasta (brown rice or whole-wheat)

Rice (brown)

Tortillas (low-carb, whole-grain, spelt, or Ezekiel)

Condiments and Spices:

Apple-cider vinegar

Baking powder

Baking soda

Barbecue sauce

Cocoa powder

Coconut flakes (unsweetened)

Coconut oil

Curry powder

Dark chocolate chunks (70% cacao)

Fresh fruit preserves (sugar-free)

Garam masala

Maple syrup (organic)

Nutmeg

Pasta sauce (organic)

Pico de gallo

Red chili flakes

Rosemary (dried)

Soy sauce (low-sodium)

Tomato sauce (organic)

Turmeric

Vegetable stock

WEEK 2 RECIPES

DAY 8

CHOCOLATE STRAWBERRY SHAKE

1 scoop chocolate whey protein powder
4 ounces unsweetened chocolate almond milk
4 ounces water
1 scoop Abadi Beverly Hills Fiber Blend or chocolate whey protein powder
¾ cup frozen strawberries

Combine all ingredients in blender, and blend until smooth.

SALMON NICOISE SALAD

3 small red potatoes with skin on
½ cup fresh green beans
¼ cup balsamic vinegar
2 teaspoons olive oil
2 teaspoons Dijon mustard
1 clove garlic, crushed
1 teaspoon grapeseed oil
⅛ teaspoon salt
5 ounces raw salmon filet, preferably wild
1 lemon
1 hard-boiled egg
1 small tomato, chopped
1 cup mixed greens

Boil potatoes and steam green beans. Meanwhile, in small bowl, whisk together vinegar, olive oil, mustard, and garlic to create dressing. Set aside.

Heat skillet with grapeseed oil over medium-high heat. Season salmon with salt. Add salmon, skin side down, and cook for 2 minutes. Add ¼ inch of water to skillet, and squeeze lemon juice onto salmon. Cover and simmer until salmon is opaque, about 10–12 minutes.

When potatoes are done, slice into quarters. Slice hard-boiled egg into quarters. Assemble potatoes, beans, salmon, egg, and tomatoes on a bed of mixed greens and top with dressing.

BROILED TOP SIRLOIN

One 4-ounce top sirloin steak, 1- to 2-inches thick
⅛ teaspoon salt
Black pepper, coarsely ground, to taste
1 teaspoon butter
⅛ teaspoon chili powder

Preheat the oven to broil. Sprinkle sirloin with salt, black pepper, and chili powder, and place on broiler rack. Spread ½ teaspoon butter on sirloin and broil for about 4 minutes. Turn sirloin and spread the remainder of butter on the other side. Broil to preferred doneness and serve.

ROASTED BUTTERNUT SQUASH

1 cup peeled, cubed butternut squash
2 teaspoons grapeseed oil
¼ teaspoon sea salt
Dash of curry powder

Preheat oven to 425 degrees. Toss squash with oil and spices. Spread mixture evenly on baking sheet and roast for 20 minutes or until tender.

<u>DAY 9</u>

PROTEIN PANCAKES

1/3 cup gluten-free pancake mix
1/3 cup vanilla whey protein powder
1/3 cup ground flaxmeal
¼ cup unsweetened vanilla almond milk
2 eggs
½ teaspoon cinnamon
1 teaspoon xylitol
1 teaspoon olive oil or grapeseed oil
4 teaspoons organic maple syrup

In a medium bowl, combine pancake mix, whey powder, and flaxmeal. Add almond milk slowly, stirring until batter becomes moist. Add eggs, cinnamon, and xylitol and mix well. Place medium skillet over medium-high heat and add oil. Pour four portions of approximately ¼ cup pancake batter onto the skillet, making 4 pancakes. Remove from skillet, and top each pancake with 1 teaspoon maple syrup. Makes 2 servings.

CHOCOLATE PUDDING

6 ounces unsweetened chocolate almond milk
1 medium avocado
1–2 heaping teaspoons ground flaxmeal
1 heaping tablespoon cocoa powder
2 scoops chocolate whey protein powder
1 tablespoon xylitol

Combine all ingredients in blender. Blend until smooth. Note: You may need more flax or avocado to reach desired thickness. Refrigerate 1 hour before serving.

MEDITERRANEAN CHICKEN BURGER

8 ounces white ground chicken
¼ teaspoon dried oregano
¼ teaspoon dried basil
4 sundried tomatoes, chopped
1 clove garlic, crushed
2 teaspoons feta cheese
1 hamburger bun (Ezekiel or whole-grain)

Mix first six ingredients and mold into 2 patties. Cook on stovetop in a skillet until cooked through, about 4 minutes on each side. Serve on ½ burger bun. Makes 2 servings.

ITALIAN TURKEY SAUSAGE STIR-FRY

½ cup brown rice
1 cup chopped peppers (red and yellow)
½ cup white onion, chopped
⅛ teaspoon salt
1 teaspoon grapeseed oil
2 spicy turkey sausage links (approximately 4 ounces), chopped

Cook rice according to package directions. Sauté peppers, onions, and salt in oil until softened, about 2 minutes. Add sausage and cook until done. Serve over rice.

DAY 10

VEGGIE OMELET

2 whole eggs
2 egg whites
1 cup fresh spinach leaves
2 teaspoons feta cheese
2 tablespoons jarred chunky salsa
2 teaspoons chopped mango

Fold in spinach leaves while preparing omelet. After cooked, crumble feta on top and add salsa and mango.

ORIENTAL CHICKEN WRAP

½ cup apple-cider vinegar
1 teaspoon olive oil
1 teaspoon soy sauce
⅛ teaspoon xylitol powder
⅛ teaspoon red chili flakes
4 ounces grilled chicken
¼ cup mandarin oranges (optional)
1 cup mixed greens
1 tortilla (low-carb, whole-grain, spelt, or Ezekiel)

Combine vinegar, olive oil, soy sauce, xylitol, and chili flakes to make dressing. In large bowl, mix chicken, oranges (if using), and greens. Add dressing and toss until mixed. Allow to marinate for 15 minutes. Wrap mixture in tortilla.

TURKEY BLACK BEAN CHILI

8 ounces ground white turkey meat
1 teaspoon grapeseed oil
¼ teaspoon chili powder
¼ teaspoon dried basil
¼ teaspoon dried oregano
¼ teaspoon garlic powder
2 tablespoons red onion
2 tablespoons chopped red pepper
2 teaspoons barbecue sauce
One 16-ounce can organic black beans, rinsed
One 16-ounce can organic tomato sauce

Brown turkey in skillet with grapeseed oil, spices, onion, and pepper. Transfer mixture to a large pot and add barbecue sauce, beans, and tomato sauce. Let simmer for 25 minutes. Makes 2 servings.

DAY 11

BUTTERNUT SQUASH SOUP

1 small red onion
1 stalk celery
1 tablespoon grapeseed oil
1 large butternut squash, cut and peeled about 3 cups total
⅓ teaspoon curry powder
1 pinch garam masala
¼ teaspoon sea salt
1 cup vegetable stock
⅓ cup light coconut milk

Sauté onion and celery in oil. In large pot, mix 2 cups squash with spices. Cover with stock, adding water if needed. The squash should be just barely covered with liquid. Boil mixture until squash is tender, about 20 minutes. Transfer mixture to blender, add coconut milk, and blend until smooth.

DAY 12

CHOCOLATE PROTEIN MUFFINS

½ cup ground flaxseed meal
½ cup chocolate whey protein powder
2 teaspoons baking powder
1 teaspoon baking soda
1 teaspoon cinnamon
3 tablespoons cocoa powder
⅓ cup xylitol powder
½ teaspoon salt
4 tablespoons coconut oil
2 eggs
2 teaspoons vanilla extract
1 cup zucchini, peeled and grated
1 cup ricotta cheese
½ cup organic unsweetened coconut flakes (optional)
3 tablespoons of dark chocolate chunks (70% cacao) (optional)

Preheat oven to 350 degrees. Line muffin tin with paper muffin cups. Mix flax, protein powder, baking powder, baking soda, cinnamon, cocoa powder, xylitol, and salt in a small bowl. In large bowl, mix oil, eggs, vanilla, grated zucchini, cheese, and coconut. Fold dry ingredients into liquid ingredients. Fold in chocolate chunks. Spoon into muffin tins and bake for 20–25 minutes. Makes approximately a dozen muffins.

PUMPKIN YOGURT

½ cup 2% Greek yogurt
2 teaspoons pumpkin puree
¼ teaspoon pumpkin pie spice
1 teaspoon xylitol

Mix all ingredients together.

TURKEY ROLL-UPS

4 spears asparagus
1 teaspoon cream cheese or goat cheese
4 slices of deli turkey (low-sodium)

Lightly steam asparagus. When asparagus is ready, spread cheese on turkey slices and roll one slice of turkey around each spear of asparagus.

LENTIL SOUP

1 large carrot, peeled and chopped
1 celery stalk, chopped
1 small onion, chopped
1 clove of garlic
2 cups cooked or canned lentils
1 cup vegetable stock
8 ounces canned, chopped tomatoes
¼ teaspoon turmeric
¼ teaspoon sea salt

Sauté carrot, celery, onion, and garlic. Add lentils, stock, and tomatoes. Stir in spices and allow to simmer for 30 minutes. Makes 2 servings.

VANILLA STRAWBERRY SHAKE

4 ounces light coconut milk
4 ounces water
1 scoop vanilla whey protein powder
½ cup frozen strawberries or other berries
1 tablespoon Abadi Beverly Hills Fiber Blend or ground flaxseeds

Combine all ingredients in blender and blend until smooth.

BROILED FILET MIGNON

One 4-ounce filet, 1- to 2-inches thick
⅛ teaspoon salt
⅛ teaspoon black pepper, coarsely ground
1 teaspoon butter

Preheat oven to broil. Sprinkle filet with salt and black pepper and place on broiler rack. Spread ½ teaspoon butter on filet and broil for about 8 minutes. Use remainder of butter on filet when you turn it. Broil to preferred doneness and serve.

SAUTÉED SPINACH

1 teaspoon olive oil
1 clove garlic, chopped
2 cups washed baby spinach
Pinch of salt

In skillet, heat olive oil and garlic until garlic is golden (do not overcook garlic or it will be bitter). Add spinach and 1 teaspoon of water. Stir. Cook spinach until wilted. Makes 2 servings.

ROASTED ROSEMARY POTATOES

2 large white potatoes, chopped into 1½-inch pieces
1 tablespoon grapeseed oil
1 clove of garlic, crushed
¼ teaspoon sea salt
⅓ teaspoon dried rosemary

Preheat oven to 400 degrees. Mix all ingredients together. Bake for 20 minutes. Remove, toss potatoes, and cook for 20 more minutes. Makes 4 servings.

<u>DAY 13</u>

SOUTH-OF-THE-BORDER SCRAMBLE

1 whole egg
3 egg whites
½ cup organic canned pinto beans, drained
2 teaspoons pico de gallo
2 teaspoons Cotija cheese (white Mexican cheese)
⅓ avocado
1 jalapeño, sliced (optional)

Beat eggs and eggs whites in small bowl, then add to skillet and scramble with beans. When done, serve with pico de gallo, cheese, and avocado. Add jalapeños if you like it spicy!

MINI PIZZAS

2 tablespoons pasta sauce
½ cup mixed steamed cauliflower, broccoli, and red or yellow peppers
1 Ezekiel sprouted English muffin
3 ounces grilled chicken breast, chopped into bite-sized pieces
2 teaspoons part-skim mozzarella cheese

Preheat the broiler. Pour pasta sauce and mixed vegetables into blender; puree until smooth. Cut English muffin in half and spread sauce evenly on both halves. Top with chicken and mozzarella. Place under broiler until cheese melts.

TUNA PASTA

½ cup brown-rice pasta or whole-wheat pasta
1 cup chopped broccoli
1 can chunk light tuna in water, drained
¼ teaspoon garlic powder
⅛ teaspoon red chili flakes (optional)
2 teaspoons olive oil
2 teaspoons goat cheese
1 tablespoon pasta sauce

Cook pasta and add broccoli 2 minutes before pasta is done. Drain and mix with tuna, garlic powder, and red chili flakes. Toss with olive oil, then mix in goat cheese and pasta sauce.

DAY 14

SWEET POTATO PIE PROTEIN SHAKE

4 ounces unsweetened vanilla almond milk
4 ounces cold water
½ cooked sweet potato (bake night before and chill)
¼ teaspoon ground cinnamon
¼ teaspoon ground nutmeg
1 scoop vanilla whey protein powder
1 scoop Abadi Beverly Hills Fiber Blend or an additional scoop of vanilla whey protein powder
1 teaspoon xylitol powder
4 ice cubes

Combine all ingredients in blender and blend until smooth.

WHITE BEAN DIP

2 cups white beans (canned or freshly prepared)
1 clove garlic
¼ cup olive oil
¼ teaspoon chili powder

Combine all ingredients in blender or food processor, and pulse until smooth.

CURRIED TUNA SALAD

1 can chunk light tuna in water, drained
½ teaspoon curry powder
2 teaspoons low-fat canola mayo
½ teaspoon raisins
1 cup mixed greens
1 tablespoon olive oil

Mix tuna, curry, mayo, and raisins together. Serve over mixed greens and drizzle lightly with olive oil.

ALMOND BUTTER DELIGHT

½ cup 2% Greek yogurt
1 teaspoon almond butter
½ teaspoon xylitol powder

Mix all ingredients together and serve.

SUPER SUPPER SCRAMBLE

2 whole eggs
2 egg whites
½ cup cooked mixed veggies

½ cup black beans, drained
2 teaspoons part-skim mozzarella
2 tablespoons jarred chunky salsa
2 teaspoons chopped mango

In small bowl, beat eggs and egg whites. Scramble eggs and fold in veggies, beans, and mozzarella. Top with salsa and mango and serve.

Resource Guide

Contact Information for Dr. Cwynar:
Dr. Eva Cwynar
Beverly Hills, CA
310-271-5438
www.dreva.com
www.TheFatigueSolution.com

American Academy of Sleep Medicine
Darien, IL
630 737-9700
www.aasmnet.org

American Sleep Apnea Association
Washington, DC
202-293-3650
www.sleepapnea.org

American Thyroid Association
Falls Church, VA
800-THYROID
www.thyroid.org

Center for Food Allergies
Seattle, WA
888-546-6283
www.centerforfoodallergies.com

Jason Muirbrook
Certified Personal Trainer and Nutritionist
Beverly Hills, CA
323-610-7187
www.jasonmuirbrook.com

Samantha F. Grant, CN
Hormone and Metabolism Correction
Beverly Hills, CA
310-271-5438
samfgrant.com

National Sleep Foundation
Arlington, VA
703 243-1697
www.sleepfoundation.org

Pharmacy Compounding Accreditation Board (PCAB)
Washington, DC
866-377-5104
www.pcab.info

SpectraCell Laboratories, Inc.
(Telomere and other Diagnostic Tests)
Houston, TX
800-227-5227
www.spectracell.com

Pathway Genomics
(Genetic Testing; Pathway Fit Test)
San Diego CA,
877-505-7374
www.pathway.com

Genova Diagnostics
(Various Diagnostic Tests)
Asheville, NC
800-522-4762
www.gdx.net

Sanesco International, Inc.
(Neuro-Endocrine System Testing)
Asheville, NC
866-670-5705
www.sanesco.net

Metametrix Clinical Laboratory
(Various Diagnostic Tests)
Duluth, GA
800-221-4640
www.metametrix.com

References

Chapter 1: The Quality of Your Life

Berger, M., et al. "The Expanded Biology of Serotonin." *Annual Review of Medicine* 60 (2009): 355–366.

Brizendine, Louann. *The Female Brain*. New York: Morgan Road Books, 2006.

Darnell, James, Harvey Lodish, and David Baltimore. *Molecular Cell Biology,* 3rd ed. New York: W. H. Freeman, 1996.

Helmly, Pam Machemehl. "Neurotransmitter Balancing, Implemented Properly: An Indispensable Clinical Tool." *Townsend Letter for Doctors and Patients.* Retrieved on August 8, 2010, at http://findarticles.com/p/articles/mi_m0ISW/is_282/ai_n19170309.

Stanimirovic, Danica, and Kei Satoh. "Inflammatory Mediators of Cerebral Endothelium: A Role in Ischemic Brain Inflammation." *Brain Pathology* 10 (2000): 113–126.

Sugaya, Kiminobu, Tolga Uz, et al. "New Anti-inflammatory Treatment Strategy in Alzheimer's Disease." *The Japanese Journal of Pharmacology* 82, no. 2 (2000): 85–94.

Chapter 2: Step #1: Feed Your Energy Furnace

American Heart Association. "Omega-6 Fatty Acids: Make Them Part of Heart-Healthy Eating, New Recommendations Say." *ScienceDaily.* February 2009. Retrieved on June 20, 2010, from http://www.sciencedaily.com/releases/2009/01/090126173725.htm.

Basciano, H., et al. "Fructose, Insulin Resistance, and Metabolic Dyslipidemia." *Nutrition and Metabolism* 2, no. 1 (2005): 5.

Beck, Melinda. "Giving Up Gluten to Lose Weight? Not So Fast." *Wall Street Journal.* August 24, 2010, D1.

Benedini, Stefano. "The Hypothalamus and Energy Balance." *Sport Sciences for Health* 5, no. 2 (2009): 45–53.

Berkson, Burt, and Arthur J. Berkson. *User's Guide to the B-Complex Vitamins.* Laguna Beach, CA: Basic Health Publications, 2005.

Costill, D. L., et al. "Nutrition for Endurance Sport: Carbohydrate and Fluid Balance." *International Journal of Sports Medicine* 1 (1980): 2–14.

Department of Health and Human Services and The Department of Agriculture.

The Dietary Guidelines for Americans. 2005. Retrieved on August 30, 2010, at http://www.health.gov/dietaryguidelines/dga2005/document/default.htm.

Egg Nutrition and Heart Disease: Eggs aren't the dietary demons they're cracked up to be. Harvard Health Publications. Retrieved on November 12, 2010, from www.health.harvard.edu/press_releases/egg-nutrition.

Elwood, P., et al. "Milk and Dairy Consumption, Diabetes and the Metabolic Syndrome: The Caerphilly Prospective Study." *Journal of Epidemiologic Community Health* 61 (2007): 695–698.

Fernstrom, J. D., et al. "Monoamines and Protein Intake: Are Control Mechanisms Designed to Monitor a Threshold Intake or a Set Point?" *Nutritional Review* 59, no. 8 (2001): S60–65.

Harras, Angela, ed. *Cancer Rates and Risks.* National Institutes of Health. 4th ed. National Cancer Institute, 1996.

Humphries, P., E. Pretorius, et al. "Direct and Indirect Effects of Aspartame on the Brain." *European Journal of Clinical Nutrition* 62 (2008): 451–462.

Johnston, Carol S., et al. "Postprandial Thermogenesis Is Increased 100% on a High-Protein, Low-Fat Diet *versus* a High-Carbohydrate, Low-Fat Diet in Healthy, Young Women." *Journal of the American College of Nutrition* 21, no. 1 (2002): 55–61.

Johnstone, Alexandra M., et al. "Effects of a High-Protein Ketogenic Diet on Hunger, Appetite, and Weight Loss in Obese Men Feeding Ad Libitum." *American Journal of Clinical Nutrition* 87, no. 1 (2008): 44–55.

Jones, D. R., et al. "Physical Quality and Composition of Retail Shell Eggs." *Poultry Science* 89 (2010): 582–587.

Kim, J. H., et al. "Efficacy of a_{s1}-Casein Hydrolysate on Stress-related Symptoms in Women." *European Journal of Clinical Nutrition* 61 (2007): 536–541.

Larson, N. S., et al. "Effect of Diet Cola on Urine Calcium Excretion." *Endocrinology* (2010): Abstract P2–198.

Long, Cheryl, et al. "Meet Real Free-Range Eggs." *Mother Earth News.* October-November 2007. Retrieved on November 10, 2009, from http://www.motherearthnews.com/Real-Food/2007-10-01/Tests-Reveal-Healthier-Eggs.aspx.

Martinez-Montemayor, M. M., et al. "Individual and Combined Soy Isoflavones Exert Differential Effects on Metastic Cancer Progression." *Clinical and Experimental Metastasis* 27, no. 7 (2010): 465–480.

Organic and Non-GMO Report. "More US Farmers Planting Non-GMO Soybeans This Year." March 2009. Retrieved on November 5, 2010, from http://www.non-gmoreport.com/articles/mar09/farmers_planting_non-gmo_soybeans.php.

Setchell, K. D., et al. "Isoflavone Content of Infant Formulas and the Metabolic Fate of These Early Phytoestrogens in Early Life." *American Journal of Clinical Nutrition* Supplement (1998): 1453S–1461S.

Shu, X. O., Y. Zheng, et al. "Soy Food Intake and Breast Cancer Survival." *Journal of the American Medical Association* 302, no. 22 (2009): 2437–2443.

Skov, A. R., et al. "Randomized Trial on Protein vs Carbohydrate in Ad Libitum Fat Reduced Diet for the Treatment of Obesity." *International Journal of Obesity* 23, no. 5 (1999): 528–536.

Taubes, Gary. "What If It's All Been a Big Fat Lie?" *The New York Times,* July 7, 2002. Retrieved on July 4, 2010, at http://www.nytimes.com/2002/07/07/magazine/what-if-it-s-all-been-a-big-fat-lie.html.

Wu, A. H., et al. "Soy Intake and Breast Cancer Risk in Singapore Chinese Health Study." *British Journal of Cancer* 99, no. 1 (2008): 196–200.

Chapter 3: Step #2: Get Your Gut in Shape

Abu-Elteen, Khaled H. "The Influence of Dietary Carbohydrates on *In Vitro* Adherence of Four Candida Species to Human Buccal Epithelial Cells." *Microbial Ecology in Health and Disease* 17, no. 3 (2005): 156–162.

Albert Einstein College of Medicine. "Probiotics May Help People Taking Antibiotics." *ScienceDaily*. Retrieved on September 15, 2010, from http://www. sciencedaily.com /releases/2008/12/081217190443.htm.

Anderson, K. E., and A. Kappas. "Dietary Regulation of Cytochrome P450." *Annual Review of Nutrition* 11 (1991): 141–167.

Anoma, O.I . "Nutrition and Health Aspects of Free Radicals and Antioxidants." *Food and Chemical Toxicology* 32, no. 7 (1994): 671–683.

Astegiano, M., et al. "Clinical Approach to Irritable Bowel Syndrome." *Minerva Gastroenterologica e Dietologica* 54, no. 3 (2008): 251–258.

Aw, T. Y., and D. P. Jones. "Nutrient Supply and Mitochondrial Function." *Annual Review of Nutrition* 9 (1989): 229–251.

Cash, D., et al. "Total costs of IBS: Employer and Managed Care Perspective." *American Journal of Managed Care* 11, 1 Suppl (2005): S7–16.

Corazziari, E., et al. "Gallstones, Cholecystectomy and Irritable Bowel Syndrome (IBS): MICOL Population-Based Study." *Digestive and Liver Disease* 40, no. 12 (2008): 944–950.

Faber, S., et al. "The Use of Probiotics in the Treatment of Irritable Bowel Syndrome: Two Case Reports." *Alternative Therapies in Health and Medicine* 11, no. 4 (2005): 60–62.

Fukudo, S., et al. "Brain-Gut Response to Stress and Cholinergic Stimulation in Irritable Bowel Syndrome. A Preliminary Study." *Journal of Clinical Gastroenterology* 17, no. 2 (1993): 133–141.

Getahun, S. M., et al. "Conversion of Glucosinolates to Isoththiocyanates in Humans after Ingestion of Cooked Watercress." *Cancer Epidemiological Biomarkers Prevention* 8, no. 5 (1999): 447–451.

Goehler, L. F., et al. "Infection-Induced Viscerosensory Signals from the Gut Enhance Anxiety: Implications for Psychoneuroimmunology." *Brain, Behavior, and Immunity* 21 (2007): 721–726.

Humphries, P., et al. "Direct and Indirect Cellular Effects of Aspartame on the Brain." *European Journal of Clinical Nutrition* 62: 451–462.

Kligler, B., et al. "Probiotics." *American Family Physician* 78, no. 9 (2008): 1073–1078.

Lall, S. B., et al. "Role of Nutrition in Toxic Injury." *Indian Journal of Experimental Biology* 37, no. 2 (1999): 109–116.

Liska, D. J. "The Role of Detoxification in the Prevention of Chronic Degenerative Diseases." *Applied Nutritional Science Reports* (2002).

Logan, A., et al. "Chronic Fatigue syndrome: Lactic Acid Bacteria May Be of Therapeutic Value." *Medical Hypotheses* 60 (2003): 915–923.

Lyte, M., et al. "Anxiogenic Effect of Subclinical Bacterial Infection in Mice in the

Absence of Overt Immune Activation." *Physiology & Behavior* 65 (1998): 63–68.

Orr, W. C., et al. "Sleep and Gastric Function in Irritable Bowel Syndrome: Derailing the Brain-Gut Axis." *Gut* 41, no. 3 (1997): 390–393.

Quigley. E. M. "The Efficacy of Probiotics in IBS." *Journal of Clinical Gastroenterology* 42, Suppl. 2 (2008): S85–90.

Quigley, E. M., et al. "Irritable Bowel Syndrome: The Burden and Unmet Needs in Europe." *Digestive and Liver Disease* 38, no. 10 (2006): 717–723.

Rao, A., et al. "A Randomized, Double-Blind, Placebo-Controlled Pilot Study of a Probiotics in Emotional Symptoms of Chronic Fatigue Syndrome." *Gut Pathology* 1 (2009): 6.

Roundtree, Robert. Proven Therapeutic Benefits of High Quality Probiotics. *Applied Nutritional Science Reports*. 2002.

Shanre, Denk, et al. "Evaluation of a Detoxification Regimen for Fat Stored Zenobiotics." *Medical Hypotheses* 1982 (2009): 9.

Sullivan, A., et al. "Effect of Supplement with Lactic-Acid Producing Bacteria on Fatigue and Physical Activity in Patients with Chronic Fatigue Syndrome." *Nutrition Journal* 8 (2009): 4.

Whitehead, W. E., et al. "Systematic Review of the Comorbidity of Irritable Bowel Syndrome with Other Disorders: What Are the Causes and Implications?" *Gastroenterology* 122, no. 4 (2002): 1140–1156.

Williams, S. N., et al. "Comparative Studies on the Effects of Green Tea Extracts and Individual Tea Catechins on Human CYP1A Gene Expressions." *Chemico-Biological Interactions* 128, no. 3 (2000): 211–229.

Chapter 4: Step #3:
Improve Your Sleep and Reduce Your Stress

Allen, K., et al. "Cardiovascular Reactivity and the Presence of Pets, Friends, and Spouses: The Truth about Cats and Dogs." *Psychosomatic Medicine* 64 (2002): 727–739.

Altun, A., et al. "Melatonin: Therapeutic and Clinical Utilization." *International Journal of Clinical Practice* 61, no. 5 (2007): 835–845.

Banks, S., et al. "Behavioral and Physiological Consequences of Sleep Restriction." *Journal of Clinical Sleep Medicine* 3, no. 5 (2007): 519–528.

Banks, S., et al. "Neurobehavioral Dynamics Following Chronic Sleep Restriction: Dose-Response Effects of One Night for Recovery." *Sleep* 33 (2010): 8.

Brzezinski, A., et al. "Effects of Exogenous Melatonin on Sleep: A Meta-Analysis." *Sleep Medicine Reviews* 9 (2005): 41.

Buscemi, N., et al. "Efficacy and Safety of Exogenous Melatonin for Secondary Sleep Disorders and Sleep Disorders Accompanying Sleep Restriction: Meta-Analysis." *British Medical Journal* 332, no. 7538 (2006): 385–393.

CDC. "Perceived Insufficient Rest or Sleep Among Adults—United States, 2008." *Morbidity and Mortality Weekly Report* 58, no. 42 (2008): 1179.

Epel, E., et al. "Accelerated Telomere Shortening in Response to Life Stress." *Proceedings of the National Academy of Sciences of the United States of America.* 2004. Retrieved on October 1, 2010, from http://www.pnas.org/cgi/content/abstract/0407162101v1.

Field, T., et al. "Cortisol Decreases and Serotonin and Dopamine Increase Following Massage Therapy." *International Journal of Neuroscience* 115 (2005): 1397–1413.

Fonken, Laura K., et al. "Light at Night Increases Body Mass by Shifting the Time of Food Intake." *Proceedings of the National Academy of Science* 107, no. 43 (2010): 18664–18669; published ahead of print October 11, 2010, doi:10.1073/pnas.100873410.

Heriza, Nirmala. *Dr. Yoga: A Complete Guide to the Medical Benefits of Yoga.* New York: Penguin Tarcher, 2004.

Institute of Medicine. "Sleep Disorders and Sleep Deprivation: An Unmet Public Health Problem." *The National Academies Press.* 2006. Retrieved on November 2, 2010, from http://www.iom.edu/Reports/2006/Sleep-Disorders-and-Sleep-Deprivation-An-Unmet-Public-Health-Problem.aspx.

Kimura, K., et al. "L-theanine Reduces Psychological and Physiological Stress Responses." *Biological Psychology* 74, no. 1 (2007): 39–45.

Lacka, Leon, et al. "The Relationship between Insomnia and Body Temperatures." *Sleep Medicine Reviews* 12, no. 4 (2008): 307–317.

Miller, Michael, et al. "Divergent Effects of Joyful and Anxiety-Provoking Music on Endothelial Vasoreactivity." *Psychosomatic Medicine* 72 (2010): 354–356.

Mishra, L. C., et al. "Scientific Basis for the Therapeutic Use of Withania Somnifera (Ashwaganda): A Review." *Alternative Medicine Review* 5, no. 4 (2000): 334–346.

Murphy, P. J., et al. "Sex Hormones, Sleep, and Core Body Temperature in Older Postmenopausal Women." *Sleep* 30, no. 12 (2007): 1788–1794.

Olsson, E. M., et al. "A Randomised, Double-Blind, Placebo-Controlled, Parallel-Group Study of the Standardised Extract shr-5 of the Roots of Rhodiola Rosea in the Treatment of Subjects with Stress-Related Fatigue." *Planta Medica* 75, no. 2 (2009): 105–112.

Reidun, Ursin. "The Effects of 5-hydroxytryptophan and l-tryptophan on Wakefulness and Sleep Patterns in the Cat." *Brain Research* 106, no. 1 (1976): 105–115.

Schoenborn, C. A., et al. "Sleep Duration as a Correlate of Smoking, Alcohol Use, Leisure-Time Physical Inactivity, and Obesity among Adults: United States, 2004–2006." Retrieved on October 2, 2010, from http://www.cdc.gov/nchs/data/hestat/sleep04-06/sleep04-06.pdf.

Streeter, C. C., et al. "Yoga Asana Sessions Increase Brain GABA Levels: A Pilot Study." *Journal of Complementary Medicine* 13, no. 4 (2007): 419–426.

Van Couter, E., et al. "Impact of Sleep and Sleep Loss on Neuroendocrine and Metabolic Function." *Hormone Research* 67 (2007): 2–9.

Vgontzas, A., et al. "Chronic Insomnia Is Associated with Nyctohemeral Activation of the Hypothalamic-Pituitary-Adrenal axis: Clinical Implications." 2001. Retrieved on September 9, 2009, from http://jcem.endojournals.org/cgi/content/abstract/86/8/3787.

Wurtman, R. J., and J. J. Wurtman. "Brain Serotonin, Carbohydrate-Craving, Obesity and Depression." *Obesity Research* 3 Suppl. 4 (1995): 477S–480S.

Wyatt, R. J., et al. "Effects of 5-hydroxytryptophan on the Sleep of Normal Human Subjects." *Electroencephalography and Clinical Neurophysiology* 30, no. 6 (1971): 505–509.

Youngsoo, Kim, et al. "Repeated Sleep Restriction in Rats Leads to Homeostatic and Allostatic Responses During Recovery Sleep." *Proceedings of the National Academy of Sciences* 104, no. 25 (2007): 10697–10702.

Chapter 5: Step #4:
Supercharge Your Sexuality

Abramov, L. A. "Sexual Life and Sexual Frigidity among Women Developing Acute Myocardial Infarction." *Psychosomatic Medicine* 38 (1976): 418–425.

Amen, Daniel, G. *Sex on the Brain: 12 Lessons to Enhance Your Love Life*. New York: Three Rivers Press, 2008, 77.

Auborn, K. J., et al. "Indole-3-carbinol Is a Negative Regulator of Estrogen." *Journal of Nutrition* 133,Suppl. 7 (2003): 2470S–2475S.

Bergner, Daniel. "Women Who Want to Want." *The New York Times*. November 29, 2009. Retrieved on December 17, 2009, from: http://www.nytimes.com/2009/11/29/magazine/29sex-t.html?_r=1&scp=1&sq=women%20who%20want%20to%20want&st=cse.

Birch, Robert W., et al. *Pathways to Pleasure: A Woman's Guide to Orgasm*. Howard, OH: PEC Publishing, 2000.

Braunstein, Glen. "Safety and Efficacy of a Testosterone Patch for the Treatment of Hypoactive Sexual Desire Disorder in Surgically Menopausal Women: A Randomized, Placebo-Controlled Trial." *Archives of Internal Medicine* 165 (2005): 1582–1589.

Clayton, Anita H., et al. "Prevalence of Sexual Dysfunction among Newer Antidepressants." *Journal of Clinical Psychiatry* 63 (2002): 357–366.

Danielou, Alain, trans. *The Complete Kama Sutra: The First Unabridged Modern Translation of the Classic Indian Text [Unabridged]*. Manchester, VT: Inner Traditions, 1993.

Dunn, L. B., et al. "Does Estrogen Prevent Skin Aging? Results from the First National Health and Nutrition Examination Survey (NHANES I)." *Archives of Dermatology* 133 (1997): 339–342.

Fintelman, V., et al. "Efficacy and Tolerability of a Rhodiola rosea Extract in Adults with Physical and Cognitive Deficiencies." *Advanced Therapy* 24, no. 4 (2007): 929–939.

Goldstat, R., et al. "Transdermal Testosterone Therapy Improves Well-being, Mood, and Sexual Function in Premenopausal Women." *Menopause* 10, no. 5 (2003): 390–398.

Hirsch, Alan R. *Scentsational Sex: The Secret to Using Aroma for Arousal*. New York: Element Books, 1998.

Kaunitz, A. M. "The Role of Androgens in Menopausal Hormonal Replacement." *Endocrinology and Metabolism Clinics of North America* 26 (1997): 391–397.

Kliman, Meaddough, et al. "Endometriosis, Tampons and Orgasm during Menstruation: Science, Press and Patient Organizations." *Gynecologic and Obstetric Investigation* 54 (2002): 61–62.

Levin, Roy, et al. "The Physiology of Sexual Arousal in the Human Female: A Recreational and Procreational Synthesis. " *Archives of Sexual Behavior* 11, no. 5 (2002): 405–411.

McCoy, N., and J. Matyas. "Oral Contraceptives and Sexuality in University

Women." *Archives of Sexual Behavior* 25, no. 1 (1996): 73–90.

Medline Plus Medical Encyclopedia. *Orgasmic Dysfunction.* September 2002. Retrieved on December 20, 2009, from http://www.nlm.nih.gov/medlineplus/ency/article/001953.htm.

Meissner, H. O., et al. "Use of Gelatinized Maca in Early Postmenopausal Women." *International Journal of Biomedical Science* 1, no. 1 (2005): 17–19.

Piazza, Lisa A., et. al. "Sexual Functioning in Chronically Depressed Patients Treated with SSRI Antidepressants." *American Journal of Psychiatry* 154 (1997): 1757–1759.

Roberts, Stephanie. "Fast Fung Shui for Singles: 108 Ways to Heal Your Home and Attract Romance." Woodbury, MN: Lotus Pond Press, 2002.

Ruiz-Luna, A. C., et al. "Lepidium Meyenii (Maca) Increases Litter Size in Normal Adult Female Mice." *Reproductive Biology and Endocrinology* 3, no. 1 (2005): 16.

Santoro, Nanette, et al. "Correlates of Circulating Androgens in Mid-Life Women: The Study of Women's Health Across the Nation." *Journal of Clinical Endocrinology and Metabolism* 90, no. 8 (2005): 4836–4845.

Waite, Linda, J., and Maggie Gallagher. *The Case for Marriage.* New York: Broadway, 2001, 79.

Whipple, Beverly, and Barry R. Komisaruk. "Elevation of Pain Threshold by Vaginal Stimulation in Women." *Pain* 21 (1985): 357–367.

Young, E. A., et al. "Increased Evening Activation of the Hypothalamic-Pituitary-Adrenal Axis in Depressed Patients." *Archives of General Psychiatry* 51 (1994): 701–707.

Chapter 6: Step #5: Move Your Body and Boost Your Metabolism

Adlard, P. A. "The Exercise-Induced Expression of BDNF within the Hippocampus." *Neurobiology of Aging* 26, no. 4 (2005): 511–520.

Campbell, Denis. "Gyms Now Offer 'Passive Exercise' Machine That's No Sweat." *The Observer.* September 7, 2003. Retrieved on July 23, 2009, from http://www.guardian.co.uk/uk/2003/sep/07/deniscampbell.theobserver.

European Association for the Study of Obesity. "Vibration Machines May Aid Weight Loss and Trim Abdominal Fat." *Science Daily.* May 8, 2009. Retrieved on October 5, 2010, from http://www.sciencedaily.com/releases/2009/05/090508045323.htm.

———. "Increased Food Intake Alone Explains Rise in Obesity in United States, Study Finds." *ScienceDaily.* May 8, 2009. Retrieved on October 16, 2010, from http://www.sciencedaily.com /releases/2009/05/090508045321.htm.

Levine, James A., et al. "Energy Expenditure of Nonexercise Activity." *American Journal of Clinical Nutrition,* 72, no. 6 (2000): 1451–1454.

Pel, J. J. M, et al. "Platform Accelerations of Three Different Whole-Body Vibration Devices and the Transmission of Vertical Vibrations to the Lower Limbs." *Medical Engineering and Physics* 31, no. 8 (2009): 937.

Puetz, Timothy W., and Patrick J. O'Connor. "Effects of Chronic Exercise on Feelings of Energy and Fatigue: A Quantitative Synthesis." *Psychological Bulletin* 132, no. 6 (2006): 866–876.

Puetz, Timothy W., and Sara S. Flowers. "A Randomized Controlled Trial of the Effect of Aerobic Exercise Training on Feelings of Energy and Fatigue in Sedentary Young Adults with Persistent Fatigue." *Psychotherapy and Psychosomatics* 77 (2008): 167–174.

Roberts, Susan B. "The Exercise Myth." *The Daily Beast.* May 6, 2009. Retrieved on October 1, 2010, from http://www.thedailybeast.com/blogs-and-stories/2009-o5-06/the-exercise-myth.

Chapter 7: Step #6: Check Your Thyroid

Buckwalter, J. G., et al. "Pregnancy, the Postpartum, and Steroid Hormones: Effects on Cognition and Mood." *Psychoneuroendocrinology* 124, no. 1 (1999): 581.

Canaris, Gay J., et al. "The Colorado Thyroid Disease Prevalence Study." *Archives of Internal Medicine* 160 (2000): 526–534.

CBS News, "Oprah Reveals Thyroid Trouble: Queen of Talk's Medical Problem Is Common and Under-Diagnosed." October 17, 2007. Retrieved on December 20, 2010, from http://www.cbsnews.com/stories/2007/10/17/earlyshow/health/main3377868.shtml.

Herper, Matthew. "America's Most Popular Drugs: A Narcotic Painkiller Tops Forbes' List of the Most Prescribed Medicines." *Forbes.* May 11, 2010. Retrieved on June 4, 2010, from http://www.forbes.com/2010/05/11/narcotic-painkiller-vicodin-business-healthcare-popular-drugs.html.

Hollowell, J., et al. "Iodine Nutrition in the United States. Trends and public health implications: Iodine excretion data from National Health and Nutrition Examination Surveys I and III (1971–1974 and 1988–1994)." *The Journal of Clinical Endocrinology & Metabolism* 83, no. 10 (1998): 3401–3408.

International Council for the Control of Iodine Deficiency Disorders. "How Much Iodine?" Retrieved on September 13, 2010, from http://www.iccidd.org/pages/iodine-deficiency/how-much-iodine.php.

The Lancet. "Iodine Deficiency—Way to Go Yet," 372, no. 9633 (2008): 88.

Mark, Denise. "The Thyroid Gland and Communication System Management: Balancing the HPA-T Axis." *The NeuroTransmission* 2, no. 10 (2008).

Nomura, S., et al. "Reduced Peripheral Conversion of Thyroxine to Triiodothyronine in Patients with Hepatic Cirrhosis." *Journal of Clinical Investigation* 56, no. 3 (1975): 643–652.

Patrick, L. "Iodine: Deficiency and Therapeutic Considerations." *Alternative Medicine Review* 13, no. 2 (2008): 116–127.

Pearce, Elizabeth, et al. "Breast Milk Iodine and Perchlorate Concentrations in Lactating Boston-Area Women." *The Journal of Clinical Endocrinology & Metabolism* 92, no. 5 (2007): 1673–1677.

Pennington, J. A., et al. "Iron, Zinc, Copper, Manganese, Selenium, and Iodine in Foods from the United States Total Diet Study." *Journal of Food Composition Analysis* 3, no. 2 (1990): 166–184.

Tan, Zaldy S., et al. "Thyroid Function and the Risk of Alzheimer Disease: The Framingham Study." *Archives of Internal Medicine* 168, no. 14 (2008): 1514–1520.

Utiger, Robert D. "Estrogen, Thyroxine Binding in Serum, and Thyroxine Therapy." *New England Journal of Medicine* 344, no. 23 (2001):1784–1785.

Vaidya, B., et al. "Management of Hypothyroidism in Adults." *British Medical*

Journal 337 (2008):doi:10.1136/bmj.a801.

World Health Organisation (WHO), United Nations Children's Fund (UNICEF), and International Council for the Control of Iodine Deficiency Disorders (ICCIDD). *Assessment of Iodine Deficiency Disorders and Monitoring Their Elimination: A Guide for Programme Managers*, 3rd ed. 2007.

Zimmermann, M. "Iodine Deficiency in Pregnancy and the Effects of Maternal Iodine Supplementation on the Offspring: A Review." *American Journal of Clinical Nutrition* 89, no. 2 (2009): 668S–672S.

Zimmermann, M., et al. "Iodine-Deficiency Disorders." *The Lancet* 372, no. 9645 (2008): 1251–1262.

Chapter 8: Step #7: Prepare Yourself for That Time of the Month (or That Time of Your Life)

Aetna Intelihealth. Premenstrual Syndrome (PMS). Retrieved on November 23, 2010, from http://www.intelihealth.com/IH/ihtIH/WSIH=/9339/23664.html.

Anjum, F., et al. "Attitudes Towards Menstruation among Young Women." *Pakistan Journal of Medical Sciences* 26, no. 3 (2010): 619–622.

Avis, N., et al. "A Universal Menopause Syndrome?" *American Journal of Medicine* 118, Supp 12B (2005): 37–46.

Bertone-Johnson, Elizabeth R., et al. "Calcium and Vitamin D Intake and Risk of Incident Premenstrual Syndrome." *Archives of Internal Medicine* 165 (2005): 1246–1252.

Birdsall, T. C. "5-hydroxytryptophan: A Clinically-Effective Serotonin Precursor." *Alternative Medicine Review.*; 3, no. 4 (1998): 271–280.

Chang, Yu-Ting, et al. "Study of Menstrual Attitudes and Distress among Postmenarcheal Female Students in Hualien County." *Journal of Nursing Research* 17, no. 1 (2009): 20–29.

Cleckner-Smith, C. S., et al. "Premenstrual Symptoms. Prevalence and Severity in an Adolescent Sample." *Journal of Adolescent Health* 22, no. 5 (1998): 403–408.

Doll, H., et al. Pyridoxine (Vitamin B$_6$) and the Premenstrual Syndrome: A Randomized Crossover Trial." *Journal of the Royal College of General Practitioners* 39, no. 326 (1989): 364–368.

Gianetto-Berruti, A., et al. "Premenstrual Syndrome." *Minerva Ginecologica* 54 (2002): 85–195.

Golden, Robert N., et al. "The Efficacy of Light Therapy in the Treatment of Mood Disorders: A Review and Meta-Analysis of the Evidence." *American Journal of Psychiatry* 162, no. 4 (2005): 656–662.

Goldstein, S. R. "Abnormal Uterine Bleeding." In R. S. Gibbs et al., eds., *Danforth's Obstetrics and Gynecology*, 10th ed. Philadelphia: Lippincott Williams and Wilkins, 2008, 664–671.

Grady-Weliky, T. A. "Premenstrual Dysphoric Disorder." *New England Journal of Medicine* 348, no. 5 (2003): 433–437.

He, Z., R. Chen, et al. "Treatment for Premenstrual Syndrome with Vitex Agnus Castus: A Prospective, Randomized, Multi-center Placebo Controlled Study in China." *Maturitas* 63, no. 1 (2009): 99–103.

Jancin, Bruce. "Risk of First-Ever Depression Rises during Perimenopause."

Internal Medicine News Digital Network. From the annual meeting of the American Society for Reproductive Medicine, November 19, 2010. Retrieved on November 28, 2010, from http://www.internalmedicinenews.com/news/mental-health/single-article/risk-of-first-ever-depression-rises-during-perimenopause/48d7c9dace.html.

Kaunitz, A. M. "Oral Contraceptive Use in Perimenopause." *American Journal of Obstetrics and Gynecology* 185, no. 2, Suppl. (2001): S32–S37.

Krasnic, Catherine, et al. "The Effect of Bright Light Therapy on Depression Associated with Premenstrual Dysphoric Disorder." *American Journal of Obstetrics & Gynecology, Part 1* 193, no. 3 (2005): 658–661.

Larsson, C., and J. Hallman. "Is Severity of Premenstrual Symptoms Related to Illness in the Climacteric?" *Journal of Psychosomatic Obstetrics and Gynecology* 18, no. 3 (1997): 234–243.

Martin, M., et al. "Menopause without Symptoms: The Endocrinology of Menopause among Rural Mayan Indians." *American Journal of Obstetrics and Gynecology* 168, no. 6 (1993): 1839–1843.

Melby, M. "Vasomotor Symptom Prevalence and Language of Menopause in Japan." *Menopause* 12, no. 3 (2005): 250–257.

Meyers, S. "Use of Neurotransmitter Precursors for Treatment of Depression." *Alternative Medicine Review* 5, no. 1 (2000): 64–71.

Mills, Dixie. "A Look at Menopause across Cultures." Retrieved on November 14, 2010, from http://www.womentowomen.com/menopause/menopauseacrosscultures.aspx.

Muneyyirci-Delale, O., et al. "Sex Steroid Hormone Serum Ionized Magnesium and Calcium Levels throughout the Menstrual Cycle in Women." *Fertility and Sterility* 69, no. 5 (1998): 958–962.

Natural Medicines Comprehensive Database Web site. "Evening Primrose Oil." Retrieved on December 20, 2010, from http://naturaldatabase.therapeuticresearch.com/%28X%281%29S%28tzndreqsszcdpnmspmcyi oy1%29%29/nd/Search.aspx?cs=&s=ND&pt=100&id=1006&fs=ND&search id=24725610.

Rapkin, A. "A Review of Treatment of Premenstrual Syndrome and Premenstrual Dysphoric Disorder." *Psychoneuroendocrinology* 28, 3 Suppl. (2003): S39–S53.

Rasgon, N., et al. "Neuroactive Steroid—Serotergic Interaction: Responses to Intravenous L-typrophan Challenge in Women with Premenstrual Syndrome." *European Journal of Endocrinology* 145, no. 1 (2001): 25–33.

Richards, Misty, et al. "Premenstrual Symptoms and Perimenopausal Depression." *American Journal of Psychiatry* 163 (2006): 133–137.

Sampalis, F., et al. "Evaluation of the Effects of Neptune Krill Oil on the Management of Premenstrual Syndrome and Dysmenorrhea." *Alternative Medicine Review* 8, no. 2 (2003): 171–179.

"Side Effects of Progesterone—for the Consumer." Retrieved on April 13, 2011, from http://www.drugs.com/sfx/progesterone-side-effects.html.

Singh, B. B., et al. "Incidence of Premenstrual Syndrome and Remedy Usage: A National Probability Sample Study." *Alternative Therapies in Health and Medicine* 4, no. 3 (1998): 75–79.

Umland, E. M. "Treatment Strategies for Reducing the Burden of Menopause-Associated Vasomotor Symptoms." *Journal of Managed Care Pharmacy* 14, no. 3 (2008): 514–519.

Wyatt, K. M., et al. "Poor-Quality Studies Suggest That Vitamin B₆ Use Is Beneficial in Premenstrual Syndrome." *Western Journal of Medicine* 172, no. 4 (2000): 245.

Chapter 9: Step #8: Have Yourself Tested

ARK Adrenal Recovery Kit: Patient Guide, 2nd ed. Ortho Molecular Products, Inc. Stevens Point, WI.

ARK Adrenal Recovery Kit: Physician Road Map. Ortho Molecular Products, Inc. Stevens Point, WI.

Forman, J. P., E. B. Rimm, et al. "Folate Intake and the Risk of Incident Hypertension among US Women." *Journal of the American Medical Association* 293 (2005): 320–329.

Functional Intracellular Analysis: Supplemental Information Reference Book. Houston: Spectracell Laboratories, 2009.

Riboflavin (Vitamin B2). Medline Plus. Retrieved on May 18, 2011, from http://www.nlm.nih.gov/medlineplus/druginfo/natural/957.html.

Scheinfeld, Noah. "A Review of Hormonal Therapy for Female Pattern (Androgenic) Alopecia." *Dermatology Online Journal* 14, no. 3 (2008): 1.

Thys-Jacobs, S., P. Starkey, et al. "Calcium Carbonate and the Premenstrual Syndrome: Effects on Premenstrual and Menstrual Symptoms." *American Journal of Obstetrics & Gynecology* 179, no. 2 (1998): 444–452.

Acknowledgments

To John Kohut, my supportive husband who has always encouraged me to pursue my dreams—however crazy those dreams seemed to be. You are my partner, my stability, my one and only true love. Your pride in me allows my self-confidence to push me forward. Marriage is about give and take; thank you for "giving" while I "took" to write this book.

To my parents, Dr. Lidia and Mark Cwynar. You gave me the foundation for success in life. You insisted upon education and the pursuit of curiosity, more so than any parent I have known. It paid off. You gave me the independence and security in myself to venture out to do whatever my heart desired. Your resilience in your own lives has taught me that with hard work anything is possible. I love you dearly.

To my beautiful daughters, Danielle and Nicole Kohut. Thank you for understanding all those hours that "Mommy had to write her book." Your maturity is beyond your years. This project started out to show you that you can do anything you set out to do. The key is to be passionate about it. I wrote this book hoping that in the future you pursue any dream you may have without the fear of failure. If you simply try you are already a success.

To Sharyn Kolberg—I can't begin to express my immense gratitude. You are not only a true professional, but an extraordinary writer. Your ability to organize my thoughts in order to best communicate to my readers was invaluable. You are always calm and grounded. Thank you for keeping me on track and being my reality check. You have been a pleasure.

To Patty Gift, my brilliant editor at Hay House. Thank you for believing in this project and giving me the opportunity to express myself to the women of the world. I appreciate all you contributed to this book.

To Jessica Papin, my literary agent—thank you for navigating the publishing world for me.

To Sue Steele, my guardian angel who has been by my side for too many years to mention. How many hats can Sue Steele wear? Always one more! Sue, you hold down the fort in my practice. You embrace change in such a positive way and I am always learning from you. I am truly fortunate that you are part of my life. Thank you for all you do for me.

To Russell Kamalski. Your guiding light has opened up doors that I could never have imagined, a gift that was unexpected, yet so much a part of my life now. Your knowledge and talent is unsurpassed and I am fortunate that you "dropped into my life."

To Parke Steiger, without whom this book would not have been possible. You nurtured me throughout the process, you were my friend, my confidant, my advocate, and my advisor. No one could replace you. You are an amazing human being and I have such respect for your talent and gift of branding and marketing.

To Todd Shemarya, who never had a doubt I would write this book. You gave me the push I needed, when I needed it. You supported my early aspirations without asking for anything in return. I am so thankful for your ongoing friendship.

To the individuals at Hay House, who believed in my book and helped every step of the way, including copy editor Melanie Gold, the editorial department, the design team, the sales and marketing groups, and all the others who helped create the book.

To the team that made me look and feel my best for the cover photo. Scott Barnes, my friend of many years—thank you for your creative eye and for always keeping my face fresh. You are my Michelangelo of makeup! To Dax Litto, my photographer, and Frank Galasso, my hair stylist, you both made it a pleasure to shoot the cover. I appreciate your professionalism and guidance.

To the many professional people who contributed material to this book, thank you for making it better by filling in the places where I have less expertise. You are all busy in your own professions and I am thankful that you took the time to help me.

To my staff at the office, my patients, my family members, and my friends who have heard me talk about the book for years, I thank you for giving me the input and the inspiration to keep going!

Many thanks to my patients who have been committed to me over the years and helped me to help them transform their lives from fatigue to fabulous. It was our journey together that resulted in this evidence-based project of helping those people who are not able to be treated directly by me. To those patients, be empowered by the knowledge that you have helped others to conquer their own fatigue.

About the Author

Eva Cwynar, M.D., is an endocrinologist, metabolic medicine specialist, and internist practicing in Beverly Hills, CA. Dr. Cwynar provides medical care that includes state-of-the-art testing for fatigue, metabolism, weight loss, and antiaging. Her clients include both high-profile celebrities and everyday people. She has appeared on such shows as *The Doctors, Dr. Phil, Celebrity Fit Club, You Are What You Eat, On-Air with Ryan Seacrest,* and *Jimmy Kimmel Live!*

Dr. Cwynar is on faculty at Cedars-Sinai Medical Center, serves as an assistant clinical professor of medicine at UCLA, and is world-renowned for her expertise in bio-identical hormone replacement, menopause and male menopause, thyroid function, weight loss, and overcoming fatigue. She has received numerous honors and awards, including California's Doctor of the Year and Top Thyroid Doctor of Beverly Hills.

For more information and resources, please visit www.dreava.com.

Get the "F" out of your life!

Admit it.
Fatigue may be the
most debilitating "F"
word in the English
language. We have
more tools to help.

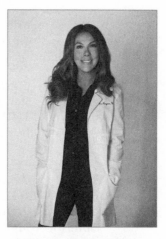

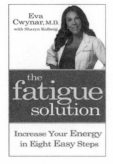

Hay House Titles of Related Interest

YOU CAN HEAL YOUR LIFE, the movie,
starring Louise L. Hay & Friends
(available as a 1-DVD program and an expanded 2-DVD set)
Watch the trailer at: **www.LouiseHayMovie.com**

THE SHIFT, the movie,
starring Dr. Wayne W. Dyer
(available as a 1-DVD program and an expanded 2-DVD set)
Watch the trailer at: **www.DyerMovie.com**

❖ ❖ ❖

*ARE YOU TIRED AND WIRED?: Your Proven 30-Day
Program for Overcoming Adrenal Fatigue and Feeling
Fantastic Again,* by Marcelle Pick, MSN, OB/GYN NP

FRIED: Why You Burn Out and How to Revive,
by Joan Z. Borysenko, Ph.D.

MOM ENERGY: A Simple Plan to Live Fully Charged,
by Ashley Koff, R.D. and Kathy Kaehler

*THE SECRET PLEASURES OF MENOPAUSE PLAYBOOK:
A Guide to Creating Vibrant Health Through Pleasure,*
by Christiane Northrup, M.D.

❖ ❖ ❖

All of the above are available at your local bookstore,
or may be ordered by contacting Hay House (see next page).

We hope you enjoyed this Hay House book. If you'd like to receive our online catalog featuring additional information on Hay House books and products, or if you'd like to find out more about the Hay Foundation, please contact:

Hay House, Inc., P.O. Box 5100, Carlsbad, CA 92018-5100
(760) 431-7695 or (800) 654-5126
(760) 431-6948 (fax) or (800) 650-5115 (fax)
www.hayhouse.com® • www.hayfoundation.org

❖ ❖ ❖

Published and distributed in Australia by: Hay House Australia Pty. Ltd., 18/36 Ralph St., Alexandria NSW 2015 • *Phone:* 612-9669-4299 *Fax:* 612-9669-4144 • www.hayhouse.com.au

Published and distributed in the United Kingdom by: Hay House UK, Ltd., 292B Kensal Rd., London W10 5BE • *Phone:* 44-20-8962-1230 *Fax:* 44-20-8962-1239 • www.hayhouse.co.uk

Published and distributed in the Republic of South Africa by: Hay House SA (Pty), Ltd., P.O. Box 990, Witkoppen 2068 • *Phone/Fax:* 27-11-467-8904 info@hayhouse.co.za • www.hayhouse.co.za

Published in India by: Hay House Publishers India, Muskaan Complex, Plot No. 3, B-2, Vasant Kunj, New Delhi 110 070 *Phone:* 91-11-4176-1620 • *Fax:* 91-11-4176-1630 • www.hayhouse.co.in

Distributed in Canada by: Raincoast, 9050 Shaughnessy St., Vancouver, B.C. V6P 6E5 • *Phone:* (604) 323-7100 • *Fax:* (604) 323-2600 www.raincoast.com

❖ ❖ ❖

Take Your Soul on a Vacation

Visit **www.HealYourLife.com®** to regroup, recharge, and reconnect with your own magnificence. Featuring blogs, mind-body-spirit news, and life-changing wisdom from Louise Hay and friends.

Visit **www.HealYourLife.com** today!